HAVE A HEALTHY
BABY

HAVE A HEALTHY BABY

DOCTOR RECOMMENDED NUTRITIONAL GUIDE & MENUS FOR BEFORE, DURING AND AFTER YOUR BABY IS BORN

LINDA PEAVY

DRAKE PUBLISHERS INC.

NEW YORK · LONDON

Published in 1977 by
Drake Publishers, Inc.
801 Second Avenue
New York, N.Y. 10017

Library of Congress Cataloging in Publication Data

Peavy, Linda.
    Have a healthy baby.

    Bibliography.
    Includes index.
    1. Pregnancy—Nutritional aspects.   2. Mothers—
Nutrition.   I. Title.   [DNLM: 1. Nutrition—In
pregnancy—Popular works.   2. Nutrition—Popular works.
3. Cookery.   4. Lactation—Popular works.   QU145 P363h]
RG559.P4   613.2   76-46807
ISBN: 0-8473-1486-3

Designed by Harold Franklin

Printed in the United States of America

ACKNOWLEDGMENTS

Undertaking a major writing project outside one's own discipline requires the help and support of experts within the chosen subject area. Because this book crossed disciplinary lines and combined two fields, nutrition and medicine, experts from both fields were consulted. Andrea Pagenkopf, Ph.D. in Nutrition and Nutrition Consultant for the State of Montana's Extension Service, provided invaluable aid in suggesting references and in carefully editing the manuscript. Sharon Burkhalter, RN and former instructor in prenatal classes, provided guidance in the medical areas covered by the book. Dr. George Carson, pedodontist, provided assistance in matters related to dental health. The Bozeman La Leche League provided helpful insights into the nursing mother's nutritional needs. Arleen Cannon, instructor in Lamaze childbirth classes and a member of ASPO, provided help with prenatal exercises. Thalia Smart, the mother of two sons, edited the book from her knowledgeable point of view.

The menus and recipes used in this book represent many cultures, both domestic and foreign. By sharing their favorite dishes the following friends helped to make the recipe portion of the book exciting and unique: Uma Amirtharajah, Sharon Burkhalter, Barbara Gunnin, Sherry Lithander, Winnie Martin, Donna Ogle, June Safford, Claribel Sellers, Thalia Smart, Dolly Smith. Typists Sherry Greene and Jean Julian, draftsperson Daphne Green, and babysitters Becky Livingston and Phyllis Anderson deserve a note of thanks for showing extra patience and diligence during preparation of the manuscript.

I also wish to thank my husband Howard and our children, Erica and Don, for their patience and understanding through the long months of research, writing, and editing.

To Erica and Don
the daughter and son who inspired this book
. . . and to all children-to-be

CONTENTS

HAVE A HEALTHY
BABY

PREFACE to the Mother-to-be

A new life has begun inside your body, and you want that body to provide your unborn child with all the nutrients needed for normal, healthy development. You are willing to adjust lifelong eating habits if necessary in order to create the perfect intrauterine environment, and you expect your physician to provide extensive guidance in this undertaking.

If you are lucky, your doctor may be one of the few with training in the field of nutrition. Most readily admit their lack of knowledge, since they are the products of medical schools that offered almost no nutrition education. If you ask for specific guidelines, you may be given a pamphlet that advises you to eat well but does little to explain the whys and hows of doing so.

If you are unlucky enough to have a physician who hasn't kept up on the latest research on nutritional needs of pregnant women, you may be told to gain less than twenty pounds, curtail salt intake, or take diuretics, even if none of these drastic orders is warranted. You may be shamed into dangerous crash dieting on days before "weigh-in" instead of guided toward the wise, controlled weight gain essential to the growth, development, and birth of a healthy child and to your own well-being. You may be afraid to ask basic questions if you've been told to eat a "well-balanced diet," assuming that you must be the only person who has no idea what constitutes such a diet.

But you are not alone in your ignorance of nutritional needs. Fad diets and sloppy eating habits are the rule, not the exception, and the middle-class American housewife obsessed with losing 10 pounds in 10 weeks may be nearer malnutrition than the poorest welfare recipient. Poor eating habits often begin in infancy and continue into adulthood. A young woman who has just discovered that she is pregnant may have no vitamin or mineral reserves on which to draw during the months ahead.

Nine months of optimum nutrition can't entirely make up for years of poor nutrition. Yet every woman's diet during pregnancy should meet or surpass the Recommended Daily Dietary Allowances (RDA) set forth by the Food and Nutrition Board of the National Research Council and published by the National Academy of Science. To assume that years of poor eating habits make a change in diet useless or that years of good eating habits make any change in diet unnecessary is to ignore the fact that the stresses that pregnancy places upon a woman's body create a need for increases in certain nutrients. If no increases are made, bodily stores, if present, are exhausted, and deficiency symptoms begin to show up in the mother-to-be.

Unfortunately, the deficiencies that do not show up immediately are those felt by the developing child. In fact, scientists are still debating about whether or not certain serious malformations may be related to the mother's diet. Thalidomide taught us the importance of screening the drugs that a pregnant woman takes. What will be necessary to teach us the importance of ensuring that she receives all nutrients essential to her health and to that of her unborn child?

Animal studies involving examples of severe deprivation have yielded results that, if applicable to human pregnancy, would certainly make mothers-to-be more conscious of diet. In rats cleft palates have been linked to maternal deficiency of folic acid; brain damage has been noted to result from severe protein restrictions; gross malformations were seen in fetuses from females with a specific zinc deficiency; and permanent growth stunting has been linked to underfeeding.

Research involving humans has also disclosed several alarming links between diet and birth defects. How can a pregnant woman be sure that her diet won't mean disaster for her baby?

Relax. Though severe deviation from the Recommended Daily Dietary Allowances (RDA) is likely to cause problems for mother and/or child, slight deviations give no cause for alarm. Your failure to drink an extra glass of milk last Tuesday won't cause a calcium deficiency in your child. In fact, even if you tried to create a superchild by following a superdiet far superior to that prescribed by RDA charts, it would be virtually impossible to do so. Concentrate instead on adjusting your diet to meet the National Research Council's standards for pregnant women.

Read over the reasons behind the dietary recommendations made by the Research Council's Board on Food and Nutrition and you will learn the importance of prenatal nutrition. Be sure that you understand the goals of prenatal weight management, rearranging your priorities if necessary. Study the methods of weight management to gain an understanding of the whys and hows of the diet that you will be following. Master the basics of the suggested daily food plans and the exchange method of dieting so that planning and preparing nutritious meals becomes even easier than haphazard preparation of poor meals. Note the dietary tips that help mothers-to-be to cope with problems such as nausea, heartburn, and constipation—problems that can make for a miserable nine months if ignored or handled incorrectly. Finally, try the suggested menus for mothers-to-be, choosing recipes from the ones given here or adapting your own favorite recipes to the exchange method through the simple formula.

Once you know why you are asked to include certain amounts of key items in your diet and how to make those inclusions a delicious part of your daily fare, you should find following the recommended food plans a pleasant task. If you've determined the best caloric level for your age and activity schedule, you will probably gain the currently recommended amount of 22 to 27 pounds, an amount that you'll be able to lose shortly after delivery.

Best of all, the diet that you need to follow is perfectly suited to meet the needs of your family. Your increased needs due to pregnancy can be met by making only slight additions to the family's meal, often as simple as drinking an extra glass of milk or eating a mid-morning high-protein snack.

Once your baby is born, these newly acquired habits should be kept. The tired, run-down look of a new mother can often be traced to neglect of dietary needs, not just to lack of sleep. Assuming that her baby's needs have been met, she often fails to provide for her own needs or for those of her future children. Body stores must be replenished if good health is to continue after pregnancy, especially if you plan to have additional children. If you plan to breast-feed your baby, nutritional concerns take on even more importance, since your body must once again provide for two human beings.

Surprisingly enough, breast feeding requires more extra calories than carrying the child did for those nine long months. Failure to meet the special nutritional needs of lactation may result in an unsuccessful nursing experience. In extreme cases dangerous deficiencies may occur in mother or child. Meeting those needs should be relatively simple for a mother who has followed the prescribed prenatal diet. With a few important additions, that diet becomes acceptable for the nursing mother. Furthermore, with a few adjustments this same diet can meet the needs of the nonnursing mother—whether those needs include losing a few extra pounds, gaining a few, or simply maintaining postnatal weight levels. In fact, with attention to the special needs of certain age groups a mother can continue to use this basic plan as a guide to good nutrition for her growing family.

Doing so will ensure that the daughters and sons of that family will reach adulthood in the best possible nutritional state. There will be no need for a young woman who has received such good nutritional care to worry about existing dietary deficiencies that might cause problems even before she is certain she is pregnant. She will have received a priceless legacy—good dietary habits that have kept her at optimum weight and in top physical condition, ready to take on the added stresses of pregnancy. What you do today to ensure the best possible nutritional care for your unborn child will inevitably influence all that this child becomes.

With the help of this book you can relax and enjoy the months of waiting, knowing that you have embarked on a nutritional course that will help to ensure a successful pregnancy, a healthy child, and years of wise, enjoyable eating.

PREFACE to the Professional

Obstetricians and their nurses have become increasingly aware of the importance of sound nutritional guidance for mothers-to-be. New mothers have voiced a need for reliable literature on the subject. Public health nutritionists, home economists, social workers, and other professionals working with pregnant and/or nursing women have expressed interest in the development of a handbook that outlines the nutritional needs of these women and presents meal plans and menus designed to meet those needs.

The professional will find that this book pulls together into one easily accessible volume nutritional data heretofore available only in scattered textbook chapters and journal articles. It contains well-documented evidence for the importance of nutrition, features a comprehensive discussion of weight-management goals, and presents easy-to-follow explanations of calorie, protein, vitamin, and mineral requirements for prenatal and lactation diets.

In addition it introduces the mother-to-be to an exchange diet tailored to meet her prenatal and lactation needs and shows her how this basic system can be modified to provide optimum lifetime nutrition for the entire family.

This book encourages women to seek professional help in planning their diets, for it is not intended to take the place of personal dietary counseling. As the Committee on Nutrition of the American College of Obstetricians and Gynecologists noted: "The most important factor in persuading a patient to establish sound nutritional habits before, during, and after pregnancy is continued personal encouragement by the physician and other numbers of the health care team."

As that same committee noted, "The prenatal patient represents an ideal opportunity for nutrition education which can have benefits extending far beyond her present pregnancy." This book is designed to help physicians and other professionals to take full advantage of that opportunity.

Part I

PRENATAL

NUTRITION

. . . a general state of good nutrition, which a woman *brings to her pregnancy and maintains throughout it*, provides her with optimum resources for adapting to the physiologic stress of gestation. Her fitness during pregnancy is a direct function of her past nutrition.

> Sue Rodwell Williams
> *(Nutrition and Diet Therapy*,
> C. V. Mosby Company, St. Louis, 1969)

REALIZING THE IMPORTANCE OF PRENATAL NUTRITION

> The attitude that all birth defects are simply a result of a
> genetic defect is giving way to questioning the possibility that
> many potential human heartbreaks can be prevented. The
> specific roles of nutrients are being examined as an important
> avenue for improving the health of the mother and the health
> and potential of her offspring.
>
> Fredrick J. Stare and Margaret McWilliams,
> (*Living Nutrition*, John Wiley & Sons, Inc.,
> New York, 1973)

Through the ages people of many cultures have felt special concern for the welfare of pregnant women, often expressing that concern by bringing the mother-to-be special food items intended to satisfy the unusual food cravings that she expressed. Even today husbands sometimes go to great lengths to find unusual desserts or other such delicacies in an attempt to meet the demands of pregnant wives. Unfortunately, while providing fanciful foods that contribute only to a happier emotional state, expectant parents often fail to provide the basic foods that help to ensure the development of a healthy, normal child and to improve the overall health of the mother-to-be.

Such neglect of prenatal nutritional needs isn't surprising considering the fact that the doctor upon whom a pregnant woman relies for advice may say little more to her than "Don't gain too much" or "You're ten pounds overweight" during her first visit. By making such comments obstetricians often seem to stress weight loss more than they stress the importance of sufficient weight gain through a well-balanced diet. After all, they are doctors, not specialists in nutrition.

Sadly enough, until this past decade physicians were not even knowledgeable in the area of basic nutrition, let alone specialists in the field. As Dr. Jean Mayer has observed: "Most physicians graduate from medical school with only a cursory understanding of nutrition. Consequently, when the practicing physician is confronted with a nutrition problem, he is forced to rely on pharmaceutical supplements for treatment." Until very recently most qualifying exams for obstetricians contained no questions on nutrition and pregnancy, implying that "'curing" or "correcting" was more important than preventing disorders. In an age replete with committees, the American College of Obstetricians and Gynecologists showed the ultimate disregard by failing even to appoint a committee on the subject until 1970.

Doctors routinely suggested weight gains and dietary restrictions based on turn-of-the-century practices, and women were made more conscious of the need for maintaining relatively slender figures than of the necessity for fostering optimum growth of the unborn child.

Fortunately, that opinion has changed and none too soon. The Thalidomide

21

tragedy of the late 1950s convinced the world that the fetus is not immune to outside influences and made doctors more careful about the drugs that they prescribed for pregnant women. The questions raised by the deformed offspring of the Thalidomide incident have finally broadened to include questions about the food that a pregnant woman eats.

Nutritionists such as K.U. Toverud, maintaining that the "child is nutritionally nine months old at birth," have long pointed to the importance of prenatal nutritional counseling. However, not until 1966 did the Food and Nutrition Board of the National Research Council organize a Committee on Maternal Nutrition.

The findings of that committee, published in 1970 as *Maternal Nutrition and the Course of Pregnancy,* were convincing enough to elicit immediate response from the medical profession. In December 1972 the Executive Board of the American College of Obstetricians and Gynecologists issued a policy statement urging members of its group to take seriously their responsibility in the area of nutrition, since "A woman's nutritional status before, during and after pregnancy contributes to a significant degree to the well being of both herself and her infant . . . what a woman consumes before she conceives and while she carries the fetus is of vital importance to the health of succeeding generations."

Earlier that year, almost as if pangs of conscience dictated immediate emphasis on what they had so long neglected even to mention, the American Medical Association placed identical full-page advertisements in many large newspapers and prominent weekly magazines, advertisements featuring a picture of a pregnant woman under which these words appeared: "The time to start feeding your baby right is several years before it's born."

What had fostered the concern of organizations such as the National Research Council? Why was this group eager to research a subject so long virtually neglected? A partial answer becomes apparent when one notes that as late as 1967 the United States was 13th among the nations of the world in the percentage of stillborn babies and averaged 28 maternal deaths for every 100,000 live births. Today, we have dropped down even farther and now rank only 17th. Nations that supposedly lagged behind in medicine and technology have better records of successful pregnancies.

Looking for clues that might help to explain our failure to lead or even rank well in such a vital area, scientists began to look at circumstances surrounding stillbirths and neonatal deaths. Stillborns and neonatal fatalities often shared a common trait—low birth weight. In fact, 75% of all neonatal deaths occur among the approximately 10% of babies born at a weight below 2,500 grams (5.5 pounds).

Since statistics mean more if they are translated into human lives, a closer look at 1968's record should show the importance of preventing low birth weights. In that year about 300,000 low-birth-weight infants were born, and 45,000 of them died before reaching one month of age. Forty-five thousand men and women became parents, only to lose their babies within a few months. Would some of these babies be alive today if they had weighed more at birth? Were their mothers cautioned against overeating yet not cautioned against the dangers of crash dieting or unbalanced meals?

Finding the answers to these questions meant looking back on earlier studies that had been made but ignored or taken too lightly. It meant listening to nutritionists such as Toverud, who had long been warning that: "Nutritionally the newborn infant is the result of a long series of metabolic processes within the mother, which, in turn, were the result of metabolic processes in the maternal (and paternal) body previous to pregnancy and *ad infinitum.*"

Ironically, the implications of Toverud's statement had long been recognized by livestock specialists, persons who as a matter of course saw that the diets of their expectant animals were adequate and offered appropriate supplements if necessary. Perhaps such attention to the nutritional needs of pregnant breeding animals occurred because the humans in charge of such animals were more concerned with maintaining the health of mother and offspring than with making sure that the mother did not gain too much weight. For whatever reason emphasis on the diet of breeding humans seems to have lagged behind emphasis on the diet of breeding animals.

Perhaps this lag can be explained in part by realizing that in a civilized society scientists aren't at liberty to experiment on mothers-to-be the way livestock specialists are. Naturally, when certain congenital disorders seem to be linked to diet, scientists have studied these babies and their mothers, but such examples are subject to many uncontrollable variables and cannot be given the same weight as carefully controlled laboratory studies. One such study, that of the outcome of pregnancies during the 1942 siege of Leningrad, has tended to give support to theories pointing to the importance of prenatal nutrition. Fetal mortality doubled during the 18-month seige of that city and 9% of full-term and 31% of low-birth-weight infants died before reaching six months of age.

While the near-starvation diets of many of the Leningrad mothers-to-be could hardly be deliberately simulated for the sake of science, a very early study undertaken in Canada during World War I attempted to establish whether or not diets below currently recommended standards had adverse effects on mothers and their babies. Grouping women according to their eating habits a Toronto team established two groups: one in which the women had diets that fell below normal standards and one in which the women were receiving adequate diets. In the first group a subgroup was established in which the women received food supplements from the fifth to the ninth month of pregnancy. Later obstetricians studied the pregnancies, labors, postpartum periods, and the babies. Of the women left to their usual inadequate diets, 36% were rated poor in the opinion of the obstetricians and pediatricians. Only 9% of the women whose formerly inadequate diet was supplemented during the final months of pregnancy were given ratings of poor.

Similar findings were reported in the early 1940s by Burke and her coworkers at Boston Lying-In Hospital. Mothers with diets equal to or above the dietary allowances of the National Research Council tended to have superior infants, while all stillborn, all premature, all "functionally immature," and most infants with severe congenital defects, were born to mothers whose diets were below the NRC standards.

Studies such as these were convincing enough to cause Adelle Davis, well-known popularizer of nutritional information, to write *Let's Have Healthy Children,* a book that cited dramatic findings in animal and human studies and drew upon these findings to cast fear into the heart of every pregnant woman.

While Ms. Davis did much during her lifetime to shock the American public out of its apathy concerning nutritional matters, she did not manage to impress the medical profession with her dire warnings.

Studies made during the 1950s seemed to negate the earlier findings in Toronto and Boston and to dispel the warnings of Adelle Davis. The highly touted Vanderbilt study led to an announcement that dietary intakes greater than or below National Research Council standards seemed to produce no significant differences in the outcome of pregnancies. A 1958—59 study in Scotland which included a cross section of Aberdeen's socioeconomic patterns concluded that the importance of prenatal nutrition was "inconclusive."

In the face of studies that seemed to negate the need to pursue the matter further, professionals continued to neglect the subject. Only when they were faced with the irrefutable fact that the United States was falling further behind other countries in the area of successful pregnancies and low infant-mortality rates did researchers again take seriously the matter of prenatal nutrition. Once the National Research Council's Committee on Maternal Nutrition had read in context all the papers that had so alarmed Adelle Davis plus newer ones on the subject, could the importance of prenatal nutrition no longer be ignored.

Considering the biological facts surrounding the nurturing of a baby, one marvels at how the importance of mother's diet could ever have been disregarded. In a highly selective manner the fetus draws all nutrients necessary to its growth and development from the placental stores supplied by the mother. There is no other source available, and if the mother's own diet is inadequate enough to make certain nutrients unavailable to the fetus, optimum development is not likely to occur. Furthermore, if maternal stores are present yet scant, the child may obtain enough nurtrients to survive and in some cases even thrive, while the mother's own health is jeopardized. The extent to which these generalizations may be taken is not yet known, but a look at the annotated bibliography on maternal nutrition prepared by the Committee on Maternal Nutrition of the Food and Nutrition Board, National Research Council, will show that the majority of research projects are proving the presence of strong links between prenatal diet and outcome of pregnancy.

Animal studies have shown that malnutrition during pregnancy can affect offspring on almost every level. Some studies indicate that supernutrition can produce superoffspring, but there is no indication that similar results would be obtained in experiments with humans. On the other hand, many studies have shown retarded brain development in offspring of malnourished mothers.

More than one researcher has shown that the addition of sucrose to a mother's diet may stimulate abnormal development of the offspring's metabolic system, a development that may well create a tendency to obesity. In this one area, in view of the strong links between obesity, diabetes, and heart disease, such studies strongly suggest that case histories of people with obesity, diabetes, and cardiovascular diseases should reach back to the prenatal period.

Even as one reads the above paragraphs, it is well to remember that there is a vast difference between laboratory evidence in animals and clinical observation in man. Humans rarely experience malnutrition to the degree of that seen in many laboratory experiments. Furthermore, human diets cannot be easily manipulated to exclude all traces of certain nutrients for the purpose of studying results. Few human diets are entirely devoid of one nutrient, though occasionally caloric intake is adequate enough to ensure survival while the absence of one or more vital nutrients is causing severe health problems (i.e., absence of Vitamin C causes scurvy in otherwise adequately nourished populations).

Animal studies must then be read with the understanding that they are not to be applied directly and indiscreetly to human experience. With this major admonition in mind one can appreciate the ways in which animal lab studies often provide vital information to those researching human prenatal nutrition. Unable to isolate human subjects and completely control the many variables that influence the outcome of their pregnancies, scientists have been able to deprive animals of certain nutrients and note the ways in which such deprivation affects the mother and her offspring. Unfortunately, since standardization of lab experiments is not widely practiced, one might find it difficult to weigh one lab experiment against another, each measuring the same thing yet conducted in such a different manner that meaningful comparison is all but impossible.

If animal studies are difficult to compare, human studies are even more so. Jean-Pierre Nabicht's study in Guatemala showed that the higher the caloric intake, the lower the incidence of low birth weights yet noted no significant differences between cases in which calories alone were provided and cases in which calories and protein were provided. Conversely, a recent study in Taiwan shows that children of mothers given protein, vitamins, and calories did better than those of mothers given only vitamins and calories. Do the conflicting findings prove that there is no way to perform conclusive studies of human prenatal nutrition?

Not at all, for by considering the fact that the Guatemala population, while chronically malnourished in calories, had a natural-protein intake higher than the average requirement for maintenance and tissue growth; by speculating that the Taiwan population's groups probably did not have this unusually high percentage of protein to calories, one can see that the studies might well complement, not contradict, each other. Even though the fetus may be able to adapt better to protein deficiency than to extreme caloric deficiency, the Guatemala study certainly did not disprove the importance of protein in the prenatal diet.

Obviously, interpretation of human and animal studies is difficult, even for experts in the field of nutrition and medicine. For the time being enough is known about the subject to allow a 1973 International Symposium on Maternal Nutrition and the Offspring's Development to conclude that "Malnutrition during gestation, lactation, or both has adverse effects on the offspring, both physical and mental." Low birth weight, the first item on the list and perhaps the one characteristic most often linked to inadequate prenatal nutrition, has been linked to most of the other problems named. According to the proceedings of the 1968 National Conference for the Prevention of Mental Retardation Through Improved Maternity Care, mental retardation, cerebral palsy, and several other central-nervous-system disorders were shown to become more common as birth weight falls.

In view of their findings the conference highly recommended that food supplements be supplied to low-income pregnant women, though their report also emphasized the fact that good nutrition should start at birth and continue throughout life in order to ensure successful pregnancies. Dr. Wasserman underlined this last point when he cautioned that: "proper maternal and infant care and prevention of mental retardation exist only as an integral part of continuous, comprehensive health care for all individuals, including fathers, and not solely by improving care during the 9-month period."

Certainly Dr. Wasserman is correct. No woman can completely make up for a lifetime of poor eating habits during the nine months she carries a child. In fact, during the early part of the first trimester, a time when the fetus is extremely sensitive to outside influence, most women do not yet realize that they are pregnant. If, as J.W. Millen has asserted, during that critical period of organogenesis before the 10th week of gestation, "a short period of deficiency of a modest degree may be sufficient to tip the scales of development to the wrong side, and a malformed baby be produced in consequence," then continual practice of good nutrition is the only way to ensure against deficiency during those early weeks.

We don't have all the answers or even all the right questions, yet we are at least taking seriously the role that prenatal nutrition plays in the outcome of pregnancy.

With this trend now firmly established, mothers-to-be may worry unduly about the ways in which their diets may influence their unborn children. Certainly there is nothing to be gained by a pregnant woman's worrying about poor eating habits during her own childhood or the fact that she skipped a meal one day before she realized she was pregnant. Chances are good that in most cases attention to meeting the minimum requirements of a well-balanced diet for the duration of her pregnancy will prevent any serious prenatal nutrition problems for herself and her child. Dr. Jean Mayer, formerly professor of Nutrition at Harvard and now president of Tufts University, has suggested that: "It may be ... that the influence of nutrition on pregnancy is very marked in the lower range of quantitative and qualitative intakes, with the effect showing a rapidly diminishing return as one nears the adequate level, where 'enough' is as good as (or better than) a feast."

With this opinion in mind, a pregnant woman can be confident of her ability to provide for the needs of her child by following a well-balanced diet that allows for the extra stresses pregnancy places on her body. The fact that opinions still vary as to exactly how much extra protein or vitamins an expectant mother needs should not be cause for alarm. There is much evidence to suggest that following the National Research Council's dietary recommendations for the pregnant woman will ensure ample nutrients for a successful pregnancy, assuming that no serious medical or nutritional problems already exist. For now it is enough to know that these next eight or nine months are crucial ones, for they provide the nutritional foundation of the child and mark the beginning of its nutritional history.

UNDERSTANDING THE GOALS OF PRENATAL WEIGHT MANAGEMENT

> The primary goal of weight management during gestation is to help promote a healthy pregnancy and optimal growth and development of the fetus so that the infant will be well born at full term with the best possible chance of survival. The secondary goal, and it is only secondary, is to keep the mother from accumulating excessive fat . . .
>
> Jean Mayer, Johanna T. Dwyer,
> Howard N. Jacobson, and Bobbie K. Hutchins
> (" Management of Weight in Pregnancy"
> *Post-Graduate Medicine*, July 1970)

Ironically, in the United States, inadequate prenatal nutrition is seen among middle-class women as well as among economically deprived women where it might be expected. Why does a mother-to-be with an adequate income sometimes border on malnutrition?

There are several reasons why the average diet of an expectant mother may lack essential nutrients, and a major one may be her failure to understand the goals of prenatal weight management. Frightened at the thought of becoming an overweight blimp, she listens to friends, and even doctors, warning her to gain no more than 16 to 20 pounds during pregnancy. Conscientious enough to starve herself in order to avoid becoming fat, she may never see any connection between her drastic dieting and her unborn child's becoming dangerously underweight. Such a woman has her priorities out of order. By putting slimness before everything, she takes unnecessary nutritional risk that may end in tragedy. The primary goal of weight management is one that almost every expectant mother would endorse if she but understood the importance of thinking of gaining weight in positive terms. That it is hard for her to feel positive about adding pounds is not surprising when one considers American society's obsession with slimness. Add to that obsession the well-meant but outdated advice of friends and relatives who look upon any gain above 20 pounds as proof of a woman's self-indulgence, and we see why an otherwise intelligent young woman would resort to dangerous prenatal dieting.

Relatives and friends urge weight control because they insist that doctors have always believed in keeping weight down. They are right in a way, since strict weight control was advocated by turn-of-the-century physicians who found that smaller babies posed fewer problems at time of delivery. To the general practitioner of the early years of this century, limiting the mother's prenatal weight gain meant limiting the baby's size or avoiding the necessity for a Caesarean section.

While the Caesarean section has been practiced in some form for centuries, up until fairly recent years it represented a last-resort tactic that posed extreme danger for both mother and child. Macduff's mother's C-section, made famous by Shakespeare in *Macbeth,* was apparently a success, since it saved the infant's life. Julius Caesar, the famous baby for whom the surgical procedure was named, was also saved by this drastic technique. However, neither mother survived the ordeal. Chances are that the mothers were already beyond hope before the cutting was done, and the doctors tried desperately to save at least one life. Surgery was hardly what it is today, and Shakespeare's description of Macduff's birth is probably as accurate as it is dramatic: "He was from his mother's womb untimely ripped."

Understandably, no woman in those times wanted to do anything that would result in her child's being "untimely ripped" from her womb. In fact, until very recently a C-section meant high risk for mother and infant. No wonder the early years of this century saw doctors seeking ways to prevent babies from reaching sizes that would make natural delivery impossible.

Decades of infants who were underweight at birth, products of the don't-gain-more-than-20-pounds theory, proved that C-sections could be avoided and that the doctors were right—but at what cost? Will we ever know the extent to which drastic dieting might have influenced premature births, stillbirths, and neonatal deaths? Was avoiding unduly large babies important enough to warrant a low-gain edict for all expectant mothers, especially after surgical techniques improved?

Of course, weight-gain restrictions were often set for reasons other than keeping down the baby's weight. Perhaps the most dreaded term among pregnant women for decades has been "toxemia," a condition so vague that it has earned the name "disease of theories." In the absence of satisfactory laboratory models and with the lack of accepted criteria for diagnosis the condition has remained mysterious to patients and doctors alike. A woman knows that toxemia usually spells trouble and may mean tragedy, but she knows little more.

Two stages of toxemia are usually referred to by physicians. Preeclampsia is usually suspected if, after the 20th week of pregnancy, the pregnant woman's blood pressure soars (acute hypertension), her face and hands show signs of swelling (edema), and a check of urine reveals excessive amounts of albumen (proteinuria). Headaches, blurred vision, and sudden weight gain are also signs of preeclampsia. Eclampsia, the end result of preeclampsia, includes all the earlier symptoms plus convulsions. Severe toxemia may lead to premature labor, miscarriage, or stillbirth. Babies born to mothers with toxemia are usually small for their gestation dates.

A mother's health is also jeopardized by toxemia. Statistics from 1940 show 52.2 maternal deaths due to toxemia for every 100,000 live births in the United States. By 1965 that figure had drastically improved, with only 6.2 such deaths per 100,000 live births. Heart failure and cerebral hemorrhage rank as the most serious threats to the life of a mother experiencing preeclampsia or eclampsia, but less deadly problems, such as detached retina, also give cause for alarm. Such a serious disorder deserves to be given the utmost attention of the physician responsible for the health of a pregnant woman and that of the child she carries. Since prevention of preeclampsia would certainly be the best insurance against potentially tragic toxemia, doctors have long looked for clues as to the causes of the disorder.

A study of World War I figures revealed that among European women who had scarce food supplies and resultant low weight gains during pregnancy, there was also a reduced incidence of eclampsia. Restricting weight gain seemed a logical way to prevent toxemia. During the 1920s and 1930s caloric restrictions were routinely given to pregnant women, although the relationship between toxemia and weight gain was never really proven.

Recognizing the importance of dispelling the widely accepted belief that caloric restriction is a valid means of preventing toxemia, the National Research Council's Committee on Maternal Nutrition reported in 1970 that, while a sharp weight gain after the 20th week might well indicate water retention and the onset of preeclampsia, there is "no evidence that total amount of weight gained during pregnancy has, *per se,* any causal relationship to preeclampsia."

Physicians are at last paying less attention to vague, outdated theories and more attention to concrete evidence as they seek to set intelligent guidelines for prenatal weight management. Concentrating on that first priority of helping to promote a healthy pregnancy that culminates in a healthy baby, researchers now consider the weight of various "products of pregnancy," plus or minus a few pounds as the best indicator of desirable weight gain. A look at those products quickly reveals the shortsightedness of advocating 16- to 18-pound gains.

PRODUCTS OF PREGNANCY

Products of Pregnancy	Weight of Products (pounds)	(kg)
Fetus	7.5	3.41
Placenta	1	.45
Amniotic Fluid	2	.91
Maternal stores (for lactation)	4	1.82
Uterus (weight increase)	2.5	1.14
Breast tissue (weight increase)	3	1.36
Blood volume (weight increase)	4	1.82
TOTAL	24	10.91

There is an indication that the body develops fat stores that constitute valuable energy reserves for lactation. Women who gain from 24 to 27 pounds (11 to 12.5 kg) during pregnancy develop 4 to 8 pounds (2 to 4 kg) of body fat that can be drawn upon for lactation. For the woman who chooses to breast-feed her infant, this added reserve may prove invaluable; for the woman who chooses not to breast-feed, losing the extra fat should be relatively easy.

When the maternal fat store is added to the list of products, it is easy to see why the newest medical recommendations cite 22 to 27 pounds (10 to 12 kg) as the ideal weight gain. As early as 1957 a Scottish research group reported that a total weight gain of 27.5 pounds, with an average gain of 1 pound per week in the second half of pregnancy, resulted in the lowest overall incidence of preeclampsia and low birth weight in infants. The 1970 statement of the National Research Council's Committee on Maternal Nutrition recommended an average gain of 20 to 25 pounds, with an average of 24 pounds most likely to result in better-than-average pregnancy outcome, adding that "There is no scientific justification for routine limitations of gaining weight to lower amounts."

Attention must be given to the rate at which the total recommended prenatal weight gain of 24 pounds is accumulated. If one justifies this goal on the basis of the products of pregnancy, then it seems logical to achieve a weight gain that approximates the growth of those products. Indeed, weight gain that follows a certain growth curve is fair evidence that the fetus is maturing at the expected rate. The growth curve used by most physicians reflects the weight increase expected during the various stages of gestation.

During the first trimester of pregnancy (the first three months) proper nutrients are essential, but quantitative needs do not increase, and weight gains are relatively slight. Breast-tissue increase is probably the most outwardly visible indication of the bodily changes that are occurring during this stage of pregnancy. Most authorities recommend a total gain of from 1.5 to 3 pounds during the first trimester, though there is some evidence that slightly larger gains can provide reserve nutrients to meet the heavier demands of the next two trimesters. During the first three months of pregnancy more emphasis is placed on the *quality* of the mother's food intake than on its *quantity*. From the second through the eighth weeks differentiation of major organs and tissue occurs so that at five weeks the ¼-inch embryo has a two-lobed brain, a spinal cord, and a heartbeat strong enough to be picked up by sensitive monitoring devices. By the time the third month ends, the former embryo is called a fetus and is over three inches long.

Weight gain during the second trimester (fourth through sixth month) begins to reflect the fact that the fetus is well into the period of rapid growth. Again, quality of food intake is of prime importance, and any additional calories should be high in essential nutrients. During this time the unborn child takes on sexual characteristics, ears, eyelids, lashes, brows, teeth, and toenails appear and it grows to approximately 12 inches and 1¼ pounds. A mother usually experiences the quickening or slight flutter that is her first sign of the new life that she is supporting. During this three-month period a gain of 0.8 to 1 pound per week is recommended.

That same rate of gain is advised for the final trimester of pregnancy, though an active mother may need to increase the quantity as well as the quality of her food intake in order to achieve the desired weight gain. She must not only be sure that the rapidly growing child is well nourished but also be careful not to overtax her own stores of vital nutrients. She has a big job ahead—labor, delivery, and the varied responsibilities of mothering. All require that she be in excellent health.

Following the recommended rate of gain allows a mother to establish a weight-gain pattern in line with the growth pattern observable in her body over the nine months of pregnancy. Considering all that we now know about weight of the products of pregnancy, the dangers of prenatal malnutrition, and the relationship of weight gain to toxemia, there is no reason to keep prenatal weight gain below recommended levels while there is every reason to work toward gains within the recommended ranges and consistent with the changes occurring within the body as the fetus moves toward maturity.

A woman who attempts drastic caloric cutbacks is probably omitting vital nutrients from her diet and/or relying on protein alone to see her through her pregnancy. If she succeeds in keeping weight gain abnormally low, there is a good chance that she may have a low-birth-weight infant, with resultant complications. To take such a risk is to ignore the primary goal of prenatal weight management, to help promote a healthy pregnancy and a healthy infant.

While no woman would wish to ignore that goal, most women would like to give proper attention to the secondary goal of prenatal weight management, that of "keep(ing) the mother from accumulating excessive fat, so that about a month after delivery she can return to within a few pounds of what she weighed before she became pregnant." Since this goal involves a return to prepregnancy weight, the optimum goal would be to work toward ideal weight for height at the time of conception. For overall health optimum weight at conception is important, for women who enter pregnancy at a desirable weight are more likely to have better obstetric experiences than are those who begin the nine months either under- or overweight.

If a woman is underweight (10% under standard weight for height) at the time of conception and fails to gain adequately during the first two trimesters of pregnancy, she has a high risk of delivering a premature or low-birth-weight baby. If she is obese (20% or more above ideal weight for height) at the time of conception, she increases her chances of developing hypertension and/or diabetes mellitus, two conditions that greatly complicate pregnancy. By planning ahead a woman who contemplates pregnancy in the near future can avoid beginning the nine months either over- or underweight. Using standard weight-for-height charts, she can determine her ideal weight and work to achieve it.

By increasing her caloric level through the addition of highly nutritious foods the underweight woman will not only move toward her ideal weight but will also increase her maternal stores of vital nutrients, an important bonus.

Preconception nutrition seems crucial when one realizes that many authorities believe that the fetus is particularly susceptible to dietary changes during the first 10 weeks of pregnancy. Since there is no way that a woman can know that she is pregnant in the days immediately after conception, it is easy to see why continued practice of good nutrition is the only way to ensure against deficiencies in the crucial early weeks of embryo growth.

For this reason an overweight woman (20% above standard weight for height) who wishes to reach ideal weight before conception should avoid the temptation to crash-diet or starve off pounds. To do so would be to rob her body of the nutritional stores vital for a healthy pregnancy and might well bring tragic results should starvation dieting inadvertently continue well into the early weeks of pregnancy. An overweight woman who wishes to lose excess pounds before her pregnancy should diet only under her doctor's supervision, making sure that she does not cut out vital nutrients along with excess calories.

Ironically, overweight women are often undernourished as well. Eating patterns that emphasize empty calories in the form of snacks, pastries, and candies are often lacking in foods with high concentrations of minerals, vitamins, and protein. It is possible for a woman to stuff herself with food, causing rapid and alarming increases in weight, yet be starved for vital nutrients. For this reason the obese woman who consults a doctor or nutrition counselor before she becomes pregnant will not only obtain help in losing unwanted pounds but also be led to follow a diet high in essential nutrients. Even as her body fat is lost, her body's nutritional stores are being increased to prepare her better for the stresses of pregnancy.

Best of all, there is no reason for a formerly obese woman to fear that pregnancy *per se* will make her fat again. By following the weight-management suggestions described on the following pages a woman who reaches her ideal weight through a reasonable, medically recommended diet plan carried out prior to conception should be able to add only the pounds vital to a healthy pregnancy (24-pound average), then to lose those pounds and return to ideal weight for height within a few months of delivery.

What about the woman who becomes pregnant before she reaches her ideal weight? For decades women in this situation have been advised by friends, family, and even physicians to follow strict diets to avoid gaining extra pounds. Some have found that the unborn baby's demands made losing weight easier than ever before. A good many might well have found starving themselves so easy during the morning-sickness stage of their pregnancies that they developed eating habits that made it simple to continue strict dieting throughout pregnancy. What an accomplishment: weighing less after nine months of pregnancy than one did at the time of conception!

But at what price has that accomplishment been made? Low-birth-weight babies, stillbirths, high neonatal death rates, hemorrhages, anemia, and countless other complications have been linked directly to malnutrition during pregnancy. In addition, conditions such as cerebral palsy and mental retardation become more common as birth weight falls.

Studies have indicated that small magnitudes of difference in diet supplements have proven significant in moving individuals from a status of high risk due to poor nutrition to one of adequate nutritional protection. Certainly, drastic cutbacks in nutritious foods might well move patients who began pregnancy in an adequate state of nutrition into a high-risk situation. Even a reducing diet highly touted as "medically safe" may be inadvisable during pregnancy. One such diet, the high-protein, low-carbohydrate routine, seems deceptively appropriate for the pregnant woman. After all, cutting out carbohydrates is not going to hurt anything, and adding all that protein should be good for mother and baby too. Unfortunately, drastic reductions in carbohydrates accompanied by increased protein intakes accomplish just what the diet books promise: body fat is burned as energy, and protein provides both energy and growth potential.

A mature adult's body can function quite well for some time on even the extreme examples of this regimen, but what does such a diet mean for the unborn child? Finding out has been difficult, since pregnant humans are not usually considered suitable guinea pigs for dietary experimentation. Recent legalization of abortion has made dietary studies feasible in women who plan to terminate their pregnancies for psychiatric reasons. One such study, involving voluntary fasting for three to four days at midterm of pregnancy (somewhere between weeks 16 and 22), showed a marked rise in ketone bodies as levels of glucose and insulin fell, suggesting a possible relationship between the hypoinsulinemia, increased lipolysis and ketonemia.

In simple terms the fetus, like the adult, is able to adapt itself to utilizing ketone bodies instead of glucose during maternal starvation, but use of ketone bodies as an energy substrate by fetal tissue, especially brain tissue, has been linked to congenital brain damage.

To assume that excess fat is evidence of adequate nutritional reserves to support a pregnant woman and her developing child is to risk the health of both. To put a mother-to-be on a 10- or 15-pound-total-gain (or less) regimen is to ignore the primary goal of prenatal management—optimal growth and development of the fetus.

Unfortunately, many physicians still make a great effort to impress upon a pregnant obese woman the importance of keeping down weight without warning her of the dangers of dieting during pregnancy. To offset such ill-advised counsel, the American College of Obstetricians and Gynecologists has recommended that "obese patients should receive dietary counseling emphasizing the same principles of prenatal nutrition that apply to those of normal weight. Weight reduction regiments, if indicated, should be instituted only after delivery." That same group offers the companion suggestion that "Nutritional counseling of . . . [a patient gaining excessively during pregnancy] should aim at bringing the rate of gain toward the normal rather than at marked restriction." Nonetheless, by implication if not by direct statement too many physicians are still encouraging pregnant women to take drastic steps to avoid the embarrassment of being chided for excessive weight gain.

No qualified physician would actually advocate crash dieting or the excessive use of diuretics prior to weigh-in day. The former might mean curtailing the intake of essential nutrients, and the latter might mean masking clinical symptoms important to the doctor's supervision of the pregnancy. Yet so many women are too awed by their doctors to question their orders, whether stated or implied, that physicians inadvertently continued to cause their patients to employ dangerous dietary tactics during pregnancy. By asking about the whys behind her doctor's advice a woman can gain an understanding of the reasons for his opinions on dieting and, if necessary, give him her own reasons for differing with those opinions.

Physicians are human beings, not omniscient gods. Though most try to keep abreast of the latest medical developments, busy schedules keep many from doing any intensive retraining once medical school and internship are over. As a result many are honestly misinformed in the area of weight reduction during pregnancy. Most are aware of their limitations, for as early as 1963 the American Medical Association's Council on Foods and Nutrition was lamenting the fact that "Medical education and medical practice have not kept abreast of advances in nutrition."

Just as women have had to fight for their right to practice Lamaze and other prepared-childbirth techniques and just as they have had to fight for the right to breast-feed their infants, they must often fight for the right to follow nutritional guidelines of which their physicians may be ignorant. When the facts are widely known, physicians will stop imposing strict weight-reduction diets on obese but otherwise healthy pregnant women. Until then such women must fight to protect their own health and that of their unborn children.

Rather than agreeing to strict caloric restrictions the obese woman should suggest an exercise program that will help to allieviate the backaches and leg aches that may be particularly intense in overweight pregnant women. Such exercises can also help to avoid the buildup of excess fat, fat that will make postpregnancy attempts to reach ideal weight even harder. Exercise may also be essential for women who gain excessively on diets below the 1,800- to 2,000-calorie range. Reducing caloric intake below this line makes accumulation of recommended nutrients in adequate amounts extremely difficult. Exercise can allow one to eat the recommended number of calories without the risk of excessive gain. Since lack of exercise contributes to degenerative arterial disease, obesity, and complications such as diabetes, even a woman who enters pregnancy at ideal weight for height would do well to begin an exercise program. A body with good muscle tone is a body more likely to be ready for the stresses of labor and delivery.

Of course, just as diets for nonpregnant women are not intended for pregnant ones, many exercises that are appropriate for nonpregnant women may be inappropriate for pregnant ones. She should check with her doctor before beginning an exercise program and tell him what she would like to do or ask him to recommend a suitable program. The simplest method of exercising and one of the best for overall health is walking. Some doctors recommend at least a mile a day, even in cold climates. There is little to indicate that a reasonably long walk on a cold day is detrimental, though in cases complicated by other disorders even walking may be too strenuous.

The rule of thumb seems to be to continue any exercises to which one is already accustomed. If a woman has been swimming 40 laps a day for the past two years, she shouldn't feel that she must stop this activity the moment conception occurs. If she bikes or jogs regularly, chances are that her doctor will approve of her continuing these exercises as long as she is comfortable in doing so. She should always ask his opinion and press him to give reasons for any extreme advice against exercises. Since those reasons may be entirely valid ones in her particular case, a woman cannot afford to blatantly disregard advice of this type.

Exercise is usually advised by physicians. If they are asked about specific programs, many can provide pamphlets such as the one published by New York's Maternity Center Association. Others recommend the exercises sanctioned by the International Childbirth League. By beginning the exercises early in pregnancy one should be able to improve muscle tone and reduce flab. In addition, by using muscles seldom employed except during labor and delivery these exercises are uniquely suited to prepare a woman's body for the vigorous physical activity that should be a part of the ideal childbirth procedure.

DETERMINING CURRENT NUTRITIONAL STATUS

> The nutritional welfare of the fetus does not depend solely on the diet of the mother during pregnancy . . . Particular attention should be paid to women who enter pregnancy in a poor state of nutrition and to those who have poor dietary habits.
> *(Maternal Nutrition and the Course of Pregnancy*, Committee on Maternal Nutrition, Food and Nutrition Board, National Academy of Sciences, Washington, D. C., 1970)
> 1982477

To a woman being weighed in by her obstetrician weight control may seem to be the primary interest of the doctor and his nurse. Weighing-in sessions are not just a check on a mother-to-be's figure control: their main function is to provide the doctor with invaluable information as to the unborn child's rate of growth. Unfortunately, the scales are not able to reveal the foods that were eaten to effect the growth indicated by the addition of pounds and ounces. A high-calorie diet low in essential nutrients may well go undetected, unless the doctor has made a real effort to discover his patient's eating habits.

All too often a pregnant woman's dietary concerns are dismissed with a simple "Eat well-balanced meals and take this prenatal vitamin supplement." Even if a woman checks pregnancy manuals routinely handed out by most doctors, she will find little detailed information on the subject of prenatal nutrition. If she convinces her doctor that she's really interested in the topic, he may give her a standardized diet sheet, which is too monotonous to be palatable, fails to explain the reasons behind the food choices that it recommends, and, worst of all, fails to take into account her current eating habits or her special needs.

Since any recommendations should be based on a woman's current nutritional status, a nutrition questionnaire should be answered or an eating survey of some sort should be made before dietary recommendations are prescribed. Since, in the words of one nutrition specialist, "A general state of good nutrition which a woman *brings to her pregnancy and maintains throughout it* provides her with optimum reserves for adapting to the physiologic stress of gestation," such a survey seems a logical prerequisite for an obstetrician's direction of a woman's prenatal activities.

Though the American College of Obstetricians and Gynecologists recommends obtaining a history of dietary intake at the first prenatal visit, how many obstetricians or general practitioners follow this advice? In cases in which malnutrition seems evident upon physical examination and/or blood tests or in areas where malnutrition is a widespread problem, such a history may be routinely obtained. Except under such circumstances what the woman has been eating is given even less emphasis than what she should be eating during the remaining months of pregnancy.

This lack of interest in a woman's nutritional background seems particularly unwarranted in view of the ease with which an obstetrician, his nurse, or even his receptionist could obtain all necessary information. The American College of Obstetricians and Gynecologists recommends two very simple methods, methods by which a woman can even assess her own current eating habits.

The first such check is a 24-hour recall. Starting with the last food eaten, one recalls all food consumed over the past 24 hours. Providing that the past 24-hour period has been a fairly typical one, such a survey of eating habits gives a rough indication of one's caloric intake as well as a broad idea of the nutrition content of the foods that supply those calories. A more detailed record can be obtained by keeping a diary of all foods and liquids (except water) taken over a period of about one week.

Though they give a fair indication of current dietary practices, neither of the above methods can provide a physician with information on past eating habits. In view of the fact that most professionals agree that the nutritional status of a pregnant woman depends on her entire previous experience and reflects habits, attitudes, and values formed and developed during her entire lifetime, the American College of Obstetricians and Gynecologists has suggested that a woman's nutrition should concern her doctor(s) from her birth through childhood and adolescence. Only in this way can a woman be sure that she is well nourished at the time of conception.

While this would be ideal, such advice comes too late for today's women of childbearing age. As a next-best solution the Maternal and Child Health Unit of California's Department of Health recommends the use of a nutrition questionnaire that asks questions beyond those posed by a 24-hour survey or a one-week food diary. The questionnaire in the next paragraph, adapted from the California Department of Health questionnaire, can reveal important individual differences among pregnant women, differences that may well mean that a physician or nutritional counselor must do far more than advise a "well-balanced diet" over the months of a particular pregnancy. By answering the questions and reading the explanations of the purpose behind each question a woman can assess her own current nutritional status. If she is in doubt about the meaning of her responses to some of the items on the questionnaire, a woman can ask her doctor for help. If a woman must seek help alone, she may consult a public-health nutritionist or a hospital dietician. In some cases, of course, a woman will be able to access her own nutritional situation and work to improve areas of weakness.

NUTRITION QUESTIONNAIRE

Please check the appropriate box or fill in the blank.

1. a) Before this pregnancy what was your usual weight? _____ pounds
    b) During your last pregnancy, how much weight did you gain? _____ pounds.
    c) How much weight do you expect to gain during this pregnancy? _____ pounds.
    d) Have you every had any problems with your weight? ☐ yes   ☐ no.
       If yes, what? ☐ underweight   ☐ overweight
          ☐ other _____

2. a) How would you describe your appetite?
        ☐ hearty ☐ moderate ☐ poor
    b) With this pregnancy have you experienced either of the following?
        ☐ nausea ☐ vomiting

3. a) How would you describe your eating habits?
        ☐ regular ☐ irregular

4. a) Indicate the person who does the following in your household:
        plans the meals   _____
        buys the food   _____
        prepares the food   _____
    b) How much is spent on food per week for your household?
        $ _____   ☐ don't know
    c) Indicate the types of kitchen equipment that you have in your home.
        ☐ refrigerator ☐ hot plate ☐ stove

5. a) Are you *now* taking any vitamin or mineral supplement?
        ☐ yes ☐ no
    b) Do you take any pills to control your weight? ☐ yes ☐ no
    c) Do you take diuretic (water) pills? ☐ yes ☐ no

6. a) Are you now on a diet to lose weight? ☐ yes ☐ no
    b) Are you *now* on a special diet (low salt, diabetic, gallbladder, etc.)?
        ☐ yes ☐ no
    c) If you have been on a special diet in the past, indicate what kind and
       when:
    _____

7. a) If there any food that you choose not to eat? ☐ yes ☐ no
       If yes, what food(s)? _____

    b) Is there any food that you can't eat? ☐ yes ☐ no
       If yes, what food(s)? _____

       What happens when you eat this food? _____

    c) Do you have any cravings for things such as:
        ☐ cornstarch ☐ plaster ☐ dirt or clay
        ☐ other _____

8. Do you have any of the following problems?
        ☐ constipation ☐ diarrhea

9. a) Do you smoke? ☐ yes ☐ no
    b) Do you drink any alcoholic beverages (liquor, wine, beer)?
        ☐ yes ☐ no

10. Are you receiving either of the following?
        ☐ food stamps ☐ WIC vouchers?

11. How do you want to feed your baby?
        ☐ breast-feed   ☐ evaporated-milk formula
        ☐ commercial formula   ☐ undecided

Questions 1 through 3 reveal a woman's previous weight problems, appetite, eating habits, and whether or not she has ever been on any special diet, including diets for weight-reduction purposes. Question 4 indicates whether or not financial limitations may make a well-balanced prenatal diet virtually impossible for some women. In addition, the question can bring to light food storage and preparation problems that might otherwise be ignored. If a patient answers "no" to question 10, even when question 4 shows a need for financial aid in the form of food stamps, WIC Vouchers (Women's, Infants', and Children's Program, U.S. Department of Agriculture), or other such programs, a counselor can help the pregnant woman to obtain such aid. A woman who has heretofore refused all government or other aid will often reconsider her decision when she realizes the importance of an adequate prenatal diet.

Question 5 covers three types of food-related drugs that a woman may be taking with or without a doctor's supervision. If vitamins are already being taken, especially in megavitamin quantities, routinely prescribing a prenatal multivitamin might well move the total intake of some vitamins into the toxic range. If weight-reduction pills are being taken, the doctor will most likely explain the potential dangers that such medication might pose for the fetus and advise that they be discontinued. If diuretic (water) pills are being used, the doctor will want to know why and with what regularity and will probably advise that they be discontinued during pregnancy, unless complications arise that warrant their use. Since many women don't really consider vitamins, diet pills and diuretics as "medicine," they might well fail to mention them if they were asked general questions such as "Are you currently taking medicine of any kind?" Yet since these "harmless" pills might well influence the outcome of pregnancy, being specific about their use is important.

Similarly, other questions on the California Public Health Questionnaire reveal matters not covered in a doctor's usual prenatal consultations, matters that might prove crucial to the health of mother and child. Question 7 covers the area of foods avoided and foods craved. This may seem relatively unimportant until one realizes that it may well be the only way in which a doctor can learn that his patient is a strict vegetarian. While some vegetarian diets can provide adequate nutrition for a pregnant woman, others result in nutritional inadequacies severe enough to be potentially dangerous to mother or child.

Realizing the growing numbers of vegetarians, many of whom have never thought about what special implications such a diet might have for a pregnant woman, California's Department of Public Health has prepared information keyed to the vegetarian's special needs. The first step in assessing those needs is to help a young woman to determine the type of vegetarianism that she is following.

Lacto-ovo—Although these vegetarians consume no meat, they do eat poultry, fish, milk, cheese, and eggs.

Lacto-vegetarians—This group allows no meat, poultry, fish, or eggs, but does allow milk, cheese and other dairy products.

Vegetarian—This group abstains from all animal protein foods and from all milk and milk products.

Fruitarians—Their diet is limited to raw or dried fruits, nuts, honey, and oil.

Macrobiotic—Those following a macrobiotic regimen move through a series of ten diets, starting with cereal, fruits, and vegetables and progressing to a diet of brown rice alone. Fluids are avoided as much as possible.

Obviously, several of the above diets could have serious consequences for a pregnant woman and her unborn child. If a doctor does not explain the dangers of dietary extremes such as the macrobiotic brown-rice diet, his patient may ignore his general "Eat a well-balanced diet" as just one more bit of advice from "the system." Presented with the reasons for such advice, a pregnant woman may well choose to alter her diet, at least for the remaining months of gestation.

Some vegetarian diets can supply most nutrients essential to a successful pregnancy and give added health benefits to the mother-to-be. The lacto-ovo and lacto-vegetarian diets, for instance, provide a balanced diet while discouraging the use of empty-calorie processed foods. These diets are relatively low in calories and fats, with a high polyunsaturated: saturated-fat ratio. As a result lacto-ovo vegetarians and lacto-vegetarians, who are rarely obese and usually show lower serum-cholesterol levels than nonvegetarians, have a low risk of coronary heart disease. Furthermore, their high water and fiber intake aid in the prevention of constipation and related disorders.

Nonetheless, even lacto-ovo and lacto-vegetarians may be particularly susceptible to certain protein, vitamin, and mineral deficiencies. For this reason special notes have been added to the discussions of various nutrients in this guide, which are intended to point out the vegetarian's special needs in relation to a particular nutrient. By observing these special notes lacto-ovo and lacto-vegetarians should be able to achieve satisfactory prenatal nutrition without violating the premises of their chosen diets. With supplementation the vegetarian group may also be able to meet the RDA for vital nutrients.

Recommendations for vegetarians on more restrictive diets are not included, since little can be done to make a macrobiotic diet of brown rice meet the needs of a pregnant woman and the child she carries. Various nutritionists have warned that young women who adhere to the zen macrobiotic regimen during pregnancy usually have a heavy discharge, experience fatigue, and show up with infectious diseases and muscle cramps. They lose both body fat and muscle and not infrequently have severe anemia and all the signs of hypoproteinemia.

Persons on extreme diets that are severely lacking in the nutrients recommended on the following pages must weigh the very real disadvantages of continuing the diets during pregnancy against whatever advantages they may see in pursuing such diets.

Vegetarians aren't the only people whose dietary restrictions may be noted from their answer to question 7. Ethnic and/or religious taboos may make certain foods unacceptable. Such taboos usually don't pose serious problems for a pregnant woman, since a woman who avoids pork can usually eat beef or vice versa. Nonetheless, a physician might well be able to provide valuable advice as to alternative sources of nutrients for a woman who refuses to eat more common foods that provide such nutrients. Though in their ideal state many of these ethnic and religious diets are perfectly sound, individual adaptations of the diets may be severely lacking in essential nutrients. A woman who is a member of one of these groups should make certain that her own diet does not have gaps that might allow serious dietary deficiencies to develop.

In addition to making a woman and her physician aware of the potential problems involved in the use of an unusual diet question 7 can bring to light the fact that a woman dislikes milk. Ordinarily this dislike poses no problems for an adult, but it might prove dangerous for a pregnant woman to completely avoid milk without her doctor's knowledge. Usually she does like other dairy products that are rich in calcium and other nutrients generally supplied by milk, but if none of these appeals to her, she may need to consider a calcium supplement of some sort. This is a decision for her to make with her doctor's help, but unless he knows that she doesn't like milk, it is a question that the two of them might never even discuss.

Question 7 also concerns food(s) that a woman *can't* eat and reminds a mother-to-be of certain allergies that she may have that limit her diet. She may be so accustomed to doing without the offending foods that she fails to consider the fact that omitting them might pose problems during pregnancy. For example, a woman who is allergic to tomatoes, citrus fruits, and other Vitamin-C-rich items may need to consider a supplementary source of this important vitamin. Certainly supplementation would be wiser than forcing herself to eat foods to which her body reacts adversely. She may well need her doctor's advice on this matter, and question 7 can serve as a reminder to ask for that advice.

While foods avoided are important, foods craved can prove to be equally important. Question 7 can bring to light facts that a woman might well be reluctant to bring up on her own. Craving a nonfood item such as plaster, dirt, or clay might prove too embarrassing for a woman to mention, but if she can check a box on a questionnaire, she will probably let her strange craving be known to the doctor. If she has felt ashamed of her desire for such items, just seeing the question on paper will help her to know that she must not be alone in her desire for odd substances.

Such extreme cravings; called "pica" by nutritionists, can cause serious problems, especially if eating large quantities of the nonfood item prevents a woman from eating a diet that is high in essential nutrients. Clay and cornstarch eaters tend to have low intakes of calories, calcium, iron, thiamin, and niacin. Other items on the list may cause digestive disturbances or introduce harmful bacteria or deadly lead into the body. While such cravings are often related to particular ethnic or regional backgrounds, they are not necessarily limited to them.

Question 8 provides an easy way for a patient to discuss openly problems that may be too personal for her to consider mentioning otherwise. Severe diarrhea must be dealt with immediately, lest a woman lose vital nutrients and liquids through uncontrolled bowel movements. Constipation can often be prevented through dietary changes such as increased fiber, fruits, and liquids. With the pregnant woman this disorder should usually *not* be treated by medication.

Question 9 concerns smoking and the use of alcohol, important items if one considers the fact that smoking and drinking may sometimes prevent a woman from eating the foods that she should. The American College of Obstetricians and Gynecologists has noted that "Maternal smoking, alcoholism and drug addiction are all associated with varying degrees of impairment of fetal growth, and part of the impairment may be related to nutrition inadequacy."

A highly significant association between prematurity rate and the number of cigarettes smoked has led many physicians to counsel their patients against excessive smoking during pregnancy. One study noted that fetal death rate for smokers was 15.5 per 1,000, while for nonsmokers it was 6.4 per 1,000. Such statistics led the 1968 National Conference for the Prevention of Mental Retardation Through Improved Maternity Care to advise that more study should be given to the matter.

Since 1968 other studies have borne out earlier assertions that the heavy smoker can be a high-risk maternity case. The mother is the one who must decide whether to continue smoking during pregnancy, but she may not even consider quitting unless she is made aware of the potential dangers that heavy smoking may hold for her child.

Question 11 allows a physician or dietary counselor to offer dietary advice on breast feeding and formula feeding. Since some women never consider breast feeding at all unless its advantages are brought to their attention, more women might decide to try nature's way of feeding their babies if such a question were made a part of every prenatal consultation.

Comprehensive as it is, the questionnaire still does not reveal all the important differences among pregnant women, differences that must be taken into consideration if quality nutritional counseling is to be given.

The medical-risk pregnant woman may be suffering from disorders such as hypertension, infectious disease, anemia, cardiac (heart) disease, renal (kidney) disease, diabetes mellitus, or hepetic and gastrointestinal disturbances. A pregnant woman who knows that she is a medical risk for one of the conditions listed above should ask for specific dietary advice if her physician doesn't volunteer such guidance.

The patient experiencing multiple pregnancy has nutritional needs beyond those of a woman carrying a single child. Since multiple pregnancies often go undetected until late in the gestation period, all that a woman who suspects that she might be carrying twins can do is to be sure that she follows the recommended dietary allowance program carefully. By the seventh or eighth month, if twins are detected, she will probably be given routine advice as to more rest and adequate food intake. The increased risk of iron deficiency and megaloblastic anemia that results from multiple births means that she may receive additional iron and folic-acid supplementation. Since preeclampsia (toxemia), premature labor, and fetal growth retardation all tend to be more common in multiple-birth situations, a woman should be sure that she is consuming enough quality calories to ensure sufficient gain for a multiple pregnancy as well as to supply vital nutrients.

Since the nutritional status of a woman is diminished with the increase in frequency and number of pregnancies, special counseling may be advisable for a woman who has "stairstep" children or whose second pregnancy begins within a few months of delivery of her first child. In such situations a woman has probably never replaced her own maternal stores before her body must once again nourish a developing child. Current consensus is that children be spaced no closer than two to three years, approximately the time required for maternal stores to be replenished. Risk of low-birth-weight infants, premature births, and neonatal deaths are all higher among women with pregnancies too close together and/or unusually high number of pregnancies.

There are more adolescent pregnancies in the United States than in any other developed country, and the number of live births to mothers age 17 and younger is steadily increasing. The pregnant adolescent is usually considered a high-risk patient for reasons that are fairly obvious when one considers the fact that an adolescent, especially one under age 17, does well to meet the nutritional needs of her own still-developing body, much less the special stresses brought about by pregnancy. There is a sharp increase in infant mortality for each year under 17. Teenage mothers (17 or younger) have higher percentages of low-birth-weight infants and higher neonatal, postnatal, and infant-mortality rates than do older mothers. Since adolescent pregnancies are often accidental, even if the girl is married, special emotional stresses also exist. In the case of an unwed mother these stresses are usually greatly compounded. Such a girl may neglect professional help until the final months, even hoping for miscarriage of the unwanted child. She may starve herself to avoid detection of her pregnancy for as long as possible, usually without realizing that she is endangering her own health and that of her unborn child.

Realizing the importance of expert prenatal care for the pregnant adolescent, the American College of Obstetricians and Gynecologists has noted that "it is generally believed that the increased rate of complications in adolescent pregnancy results from the stresses of pregnancy superimposed upon those of adolescence, each with its own nutritional imperative. Adolescent pregnancy demands a sophisticated program of care, an important part of which is nutritional in nature."

The nutritional needs of the pregnant adolescent are complex. Bizarre eating habits, including the consumption of excessive yet empty calories, are often seen in young pregnant girls. Iron, calcium, protein, and vitamin deficiencies are often present, sometimes due to sporadic use of crash or fad diets that rob a growing body of essential nutrients.

Pregnant adolescents sometimes fall into high-risk groupings for other reasons. A significant percentage of pregnant adolescents are underweight, a condition that often increases the likelihood of a low-birth-weight infant. High-calorie, high-quality meals and snacks are vital to the health of these girls and their babies. Obesity raises pregnancy risks for women of any age group, and 10% to 25% of adolescents are obese at the start of pregnancy. If dieting for weight-reduction purposes is dangerous for older pregnant women, it is extremely dangerous in the case of the pregnant adolescent. The seriousness of this situation caused the National Research Council's Committee on Maternal Nutrition to issue the following warning:

> When the nutritional demands of pregnancy are superimposed on those of adolescence, there should be no stringent caloric restrictions. Even for the obese young adolescent, a modest weight gain should be permitted during pregnancy, and any attempt to reduce maternal weight by caloric restriction of drugs should be postponed until after delivery. The standardized diets commonly used in prenatal clinics are especially unsuited to the special nutritional needs of the young adolescent.

Unfortunately, such standardized diets are often unsuited to the needs of other pregnant women. Only by considering a woman's long-term and immediate nutritional history; assessing her current nutritional practices as influenced by ethnic, social, religious, or economic circumstances; and assessing her current nutritional status as it relates to her physical state, age, and other important factors can one determine the prenatal diet ideally suited to meet the stresses imposed by that woman's pregnancy.

UNDERSTANDING THE NUTRITIONAL NEEDS OF PREGNANCY — ENERGY & PROTEIN

> Increased intake of protein is required during pregnancy to provide for fetal needs and to permit the required maternal physiologic adjustments of expansion of blood volume and growth of breast and uterine tissue.
>
> *Nutrition in Maternal Health Care*
> (Committee on Nutrition, American College of Obstetricians and Gynecologists, 1974)

Once a woman has understood the importance of prenatal nutrition, committed herself to attaining the goals of prenatal weight management, and assessed her current nutritional status, she is ready to study the specific components of a well-balanced diet and to learn the ways in which pregnancy increases her need for many of these components.

The accepted basis for determining the nutritional needs of various age groups in the United States is the Recommended Dietary Allowances chart published by the National Academy of Science in Washington, D.C., and compiled by the Committee on Dietary Allowances, Committee on Interpretation of the Recommended Dietary Allowances, Food and Nutrition Board of the National Research Council. Recommendations used in this book are based on the eighth revised edition (1974) of that chart.

The RDA chart is intended as a guide, not a mandate for all individuals. As stressed in the preceding chapter, individual differences must be considered before one can determine ideal prenatal nutrition. In addition to the individual differences previously discussed a woman's size and exercise pattern must be considered when using the RDA guide. Once necessary adjustments have been made and the RDA has been set for each nutrient, one should remember that all RDA listings *except calories* provide more than the minimum daily requirement for most people. Thus there is no need to try to include amounts larger than those recommended. However, since most nutrients can be tolerated in amounts exceeding the RDA by as much as two to three times, increased amounts aren't likely to cause problems. Two exceptions must be noted: very high intakes of Vitamin A and Vitamin D and of certain trace elements can be toxic. Excessive caloric intake will lead to obesity.

The built-in safeguards of RDA mean that there is no need to fear that including slightly lesser amounts of nutrients will cause severe deficiency symptoms in a woman or in the child that she is carrying. The body can conserve essential nutrients if the supply falls and can store some nutrients if an overabundance exists. Thus falling below RDA standards for one day isn't too serious, since the body makes allowances for occasional shortages. An average intake that meets RDA over a five- to eight-day period is probably adequate. Of course, habitually falling below RDA standards for a particular nutrient and the longer low intake continues, the greater the risk of deficiency becomes. One further word of warning is in order. For some people with unusual needs due to special circumstances even strict adherence to RDA standards would not ensure adequate intakes of some nutrients to prevent the occurrence of deficiency symptoms. In such cases adjustments can be made to increase certain nutrients, and supplements can be used if necessary.

Unfortunately, the use of supplements often gives both physician and patient a false sense of security. In spite of science-fiction stories in which a pill serves as a substitute for food, no such pill exists. Supplements should not be routinely instituted as a means of correcting poor food habits. Use of prenatal vitamin-mineral supplements remains widespread, yet the National Committee on Maternal Nutrition noted in its 1970 report that "Except for iron and folic acid, the routine supplementation of diets of pregnant women with vitamin and mineral preparations is of uncertain value."

Though some might argue that such supplements can do no harm if taken in excessive amounts and in combination with megavitamins (especially A, D, and C), they might very well prove harmful.

Nutritional counseling should be given regarding the heavy use of certain processed foods in the mistaken belief that these foods alone contain all one needs to meet RDA standards for a certain vitamin. Because many manufacturers of foods tend to feel that their food items must have all RDA minimum intakes in a single serving, they have fortified certain products to reach those standards. Government-required labels proclaim that a certain cereal provides 100% of an adult's Vitamin-C requirements. If this is true and if such fortification continues, a person might conceivably receive toxic dosages of Vitamin A or D by eating an entire box of cereal to which she has added milk fortified with those same vitamins. This is not to say that such products should be avoided entirely. Fortified milk, for instance, has substantially aided in the prevention of Vitamin-D deficiency and its accompanying rickets. Yet stringent regulations as to the kinds and amounts of additives should be enacted to reduce the risk of accidental overdoses of certain vitamins or minerals. Foods in their natural state do not contain a perfect balance of all nutrients. Processed foods should not attempt to do so either. Instead, they might work toward including approximately the same nutritional makeup as the traditional foods that they tend to replace in the average diet.

Labeling of foods has led manufacturers to try to make their label sound better than that of their competitors. It has also led consumers to place unwarranted confidence in the nutritional value of foods whose labels seem to promise high percentages of the eight essential nutrients (protein, five vitamins, two minerals) that must be listed. The fact that the government does not require that a manufacturer list *all* nutrients on a package label does not mean that other nutrients are not equally essential to good health. A woman who limits her intake to fortified products that promise high percentages of certain nutrients is ignoring her need for many other nutrients equally important but not listed on the label and not likely to be found in highly refined and processed products. Relying on fortified foods is as unwise as relying on vitamin-mineral preparations. Rely instead on a balanced diet that meets RDA standards and follows sound dietary principles.

To understand how to read the RDA chart, a woman need only examine it carefully. However, to simplify use of the chart in planning nutritious prenatal menus, this book features minicharts adapted from the larger one but including only the specific items being discussed. For instance, this chapter contains a chart relating to energy (calorie) needs of nonpregnant and pregnant women.

Although this guidebook emphasizes the needs of pregnant and lactating women, RDA figures can be of little use unless they are first examined in light of the needs of nonpregnant women of various ages and sizes. After all, pregnancy imposes *additional* stresses on a woman's body. In order to meet the nutritional demands that those stresses create, she must first meet the nutritional demands of her nonpregnant body. For this reason discussions of recommended daily dietary allowances of energy (calories), protein, vitamins, and minerals will include the general needs for each of these items as well as the additional needs imposed by pregnancy.

Energy

Calories, the concern of almost every weight-conscious person, have developed negative connotations over the decades. Cutting down on calories has become the cry of the nation's overweight men and women, yet few of the persons who discuss calories have more than a slight understanding of the term. To many persons, a *no*-calorie diet seems utopian, when in fact it would mean starvation and death.

The much-discussed and little-understood calorie, more correctly called a kilocalorie (1,000 calories), is merely a unit of measurement for energy, much like an ounce indicates weight or an inch indicates length or width. In this case the unit indicates the amount of energy required to raise one kilogram of water one degree centigrade. By its very definition a calorie is a unit used to describe work, output, or activity. In the human body that activity takes many forms. Physical activity, growth, lactation, metabolic processes, excretory processes, physiological and psychological stress, maintenance of body temperatures—all these activities require *energy.* Energy comes from food, and in the United States food energy is usually expressed in calories (kcal).

The National Research Council has set recommended energy allowances at the lowest value thought to be consonant with good health for the average person in a designated age group. Americans tend to be obese, partly because they are consuming the number of calories indicated for their age and sex groups without regard for the fact that their activity level may be so low that they have no need for all the calories they consume. Calories taken in excess of need are stored in unsightly, unhealthy fat deposits. If calorie intake falls too far below recommended levels, weight decreases, and, if caloric restriction is severe enough, health deteriorates.

Realizing the need for a careful and accurate assessment of caloric need, physicians have devised several methods for determining the ideal calorie level for average individuals of certain ages, sexes, heights, and weights. The best available methods have been used in compiling the RDA figures that appear below, yet the recommended caloric intakes might be too high or too low for certain women.

RECOMMENDED DAILY DIETARY ALLOWANCES OF ENERGY (CALORIES)

	Age (years)	Weight (kg)	(lbs)	Height (cm)	(feet)	Energy (kcal)	Added During Preg.
Non-pregnant	11-14	44	97	155	5'2"	2400	+300
	15-18	54	119	162	5'5"	2100	+300
	19-22	58	128	162	5'5"	2100	+300
	23-50	58	128	162	5'5"	2000	+300

One simple way for a woman to determine whether these recommendations are correct for her is to try the recommended caloric intake for at least two weeks. If weight remains steady, the intake is probably adequate but not excessive. Another way she can determine the suitability of calorie recommendations is to get a rough estimate of her usual calorie level by checking her dietary history (see chapter 3). If she has been maintaining a desirable weight on this calorie level, the level is probably fairly well suited to her needs. Of course, if a pregnant woman wishes to use either of these methods to find whether the recommended caloric intake is suitable, she must take into consideration the 300 extra calories per day required during pregnancy and the recommended weight gain for her particular stage of gestation (week or month of pregnancy).

Some helpful hints for using the RDA chart are given in the manual that accompanies that chart. First, the true energy requirement for an underweight woman must be based on her *ideal* weight, not on her actual weight. Second, an obese woman can probably maintain her current weight, adding just the recommended number of pounds per month that her pregnancy dictates, if she chooses the calorie level of her current weight. To choose the level according to her ideal weight would be to set up a weight-loss situation, which is not recommended for use during pregnancy.

More accuracy in determining caloric needs can be gained by following the recommendations outlined in *Recommended Dietary Allowances* (1974 edition), pages 27−30. A general idea of optimum calorie levels can be obtained by considering the fact that RDA standards are based on the needs of a person engaged in ordinary activites.

If height and weight vary sharply from the references in the RDA standards and/or if activities are strenuous or totally sendentary, appropriate adjustments should be made. A physician or a professional nutritionist can assist a woman in setting her optimal prenatal calorie level. Consulting an expert is probably wise if the figures derived from her own calculations differ greatly from those given on the RDA chart.

One further note is in order here. The pregnant adolescent must remember that she is still meeting her own growth needs and must take seriously the extra calories included on the RDA chart, calories that allow for her multiple needs. Pregnancy is no time to attempt weight loss. Producing a healthy child and promoting her own good health should take precedence over any desire to trim escess fat.

Once the daily caloric requirements for the nonpregnant woman have been determined, a woman must add 300 extra calories to allow for the extra stress of pregnancy. Increased cardiac and lung output plus tissue building for growth of the uterus, placenta, fetus, and breasts all require extra energy. Though the expectant mother may require more energy to carry out normal physicial activity during the final trimester of pregnancy (due to her increased size), most women exhibit marked reduction of activity during that trimester, thus making little if any extra energy necessary for normal physicial activity.

A gross energy cost of 80,000 kcal for nine months of pregnancy has been estimated, and an additional 300 kcal per day throughout pregnancy is required to meet that total energy demand. One important rule of thumb is to avoid caloric intakes that fall below 36 kcal for every kg (or 36 kcal for every 2.2 pounds) of pregnant body weight. If calorie levels fall below this point, protein must then be utilized for energy and cannot be properly utilized for the growth of mother and child.

If a woman determines that she gains too rapidly even at the lowest recommended caloric levels for a pregnant woman of her height, weight, and age, she should try increasing her exercise not further decreasing her calories. After all, RDA standards for calories represent the *lowest* intake considered desirable. To reduce calories further is to risk malnutrition or imbalance. Exercise, don't starve.

Energy Sources

Of prime importance is the fact that caloric increases should be qualitative, not just quantitative. Merely consuming the recommended number of calories provides no insurance that proper nutrition is being obtained. In fact, malnutrition can often be present in grossly overweight persons who consume large quantities of low-quality calories. Many Americans derive a large part (30% or more) of their energy from highly refined sugars, fat, and alcohol, all of which provide almost no vitamins and minerals. Others try fad diets, which lead them to cut out whole categories of foods (i.e., carbohydrates), an act that can cause severe complications for a nonpregnant woman and have tragic consequences for a pregnant woman and the child whom she is carrying. Still others eat fairly well-balanced meals yet consume empty, high-calorie snacks between meals. Such persons are likely to assume that they must cut back on caloric intake at meals, never realizing that the nibbled calories are the true culprits, especially in view of the fact that such tidbits are usually lacking in essential nutrients.

Carbohydrates, along with fats, are our most important sources of food energy. One gram of carbohydrate yields four calories; one gram of fat yields nine calories; one gram of protein yields four calories. Sugars (simple carbohydrates), starches (complex carbohydrates), and cellulose (more complex carbohydrates) are the three principal types of carbohydrates. Highly refined sugars, jams, jellies, syrups, milk, and fruits all fall into the first category.

Starches such as cereal, potatoes, flour, and rice make up the second group and largely indigestible vegetable fibers make up the third. Generally speaking, Americans are alarmingly higher in carbohydrates from the first group, especially highly refined sugars. A 60-year survey of American eating habits showed a 25% decrease in carbohydrate consumption and a 25% increase in sugar and syrup consumption.

Since highly refined sugars give little more than pure energy, they are likely to lead to nutritional problems. For instance, a weight-reduction diet based on calories alone would be unsound, for a person might choose to acquire the total daily caloric allowance in highly refined carbohydrates such as sugars and candies, a choice that would lead to malnutrition. A child who fills his calorie need through such means is likely to ignore body-building, high-protein, high-vitamin-mineral foods. More concentration on the complex carbohydrates is advised, since these products give vitamins, minerals, fiber, and even protein as well as energy.

The body needs carbohydrate as a source of energy for brain function and growth and for certain other specialized processes. After these special needs have been met, fat may be used for energy. Apparently 50 to 100 grams of digestible carbohydrate are needed per day to avoid ketosis (excessive body-protein breakdown) and other undesirable metabolic responses such as dehydration and loss of sodium. The body's storage capacity is about 1,400 kcal, or enough energy for 13 hours of very modest activity. If sufficient carbohydrates are not available for energy, energy must be obtained from dietary or body protein.

There are several widely acclaimed diets that advocate high-protein, low-carbohydrate regimens for weight reduction. Such diets depend on the fact that the body's basic energy requirements are met before any other requirements. The needs of basal metabolism (the measure of the energy produced to maintain the body at rest after a 12-hour fast) must be met if life is to continue. Deprived of all carbohydrate, the body will break down its own fatty and protein tissue in order to gain usable energy, thus causing weight loss in most individuals.

In 1974 Consumer Guide's *Rating the Diets* warned that high-protein, low-carbohydrate diets posed dangers during pregnancy, due to the fact that "Ketosis [the use of protein for energy because of the lack of carbohydrates] seems to have a harmful effect on unborn children. It may impair development of the brain of the fetus." That same publication pointed to a late 1960s study of 55,000 pregnancies in which children born of mothers who had acetonuria (a form of ketosis) had lower IQ scores than did children born of mothers without acetonuria.

In view of these facts severe caloric restriction should not be undertaken during pregnancy, particularly not severely limited intake of carbohydrates. Crash diets before weigh-ins and high-protein, low-carbohydrate diets that force the fetus to rely on ketone acids for energy might both be detrimental to fetal brain development. In spite of the many fad diets that tend to give carbohydrates a negative connotation complex carbohydrates especially are vital sources of energy.

Fats are the most concentrated source of energy, yielding nine kcal for every gram. Dietary patterns have shifted so that carbohydrates (46%) and fats (42%) are now almost equal sources of energy for the average American. Fat consumption has been on the rise, but in view of the American Heart Association's recommendation against eating an excess of saturated fatty acids, this trend may change.

The importance of fats is seen when one realizes that they serve as carriers for fat-soluble nutrients such as Vitamins A, D, E, and K. Excess calories are stored as fat in the human body in adipose cells, where they help to cushion the organs, insulate the body, and offer protection against mechanical stresses. These stores can also supply energy for certain bodily emergencies, although the central nervous system cannot use fatty acids directly as an energy source. As noted above, preformed carbohydrates are required to ensure optimum brain development in the fetus. Excess body fat from the mother cannot safely fill the energy and growth needs of the unborn child.

There are only two essential fatty acids, linoleic and arachidonic, and the second can be synthesized from the first. Linoleic acid is found in corn, cottonseed, peanut, safflower, and soybean oil but not in olive or coconut oil. Infants occasionally suffer from essential fatty-acid deficiency. In all but the most extreme cases of fat deprivation body stores seem sufficient to provide insurance against essential fatty-acid deficiency in the adult. When deficiencies do occur, they have been linked to dermatitis and impaired lipid transport.

One other energy source should be mentioned. *Alcohol* at eight kcal per gram has nearly the energy potential of fat without providing any benefits beyond pure energy. Alcohol may supply 5% to 10% of total energy for even moderate drinkers, and some persons consume as many as 1,800 kcal per day of alcohol. When alcohol provides a major portion of an adult's total calories, protein and vitamin deficiencies soon show up, especially of thiamin, niacin, and folic acid. For the pregnant woman such severe deficiencies might well be detrimental to the fetus. Alcohol is toxic in excessive amounts and can be dangerous in lesser amounts if it prevents adequate intake and/or utilization of essential nutrients. Possible ill effects of extreme alcoholic intake upon the fetus are also suspected, making excessive drinking a double threat for the pregnant woman.

As noted earlier, many Americans derive a large percentage of their energy from relatively pure sugars, fats, and alcohols. Since these items provide almost no vitamins and minerals and only a narrow spectrum of nutrients, it is easy to see why many persons are overweight yet undernourished. Calories alone are not enough. The pregnant woman must be sure that a large percentage of her energy (calories) comes from complex carbohydrates that can provide more than energy, carbohydrates that contain protein, vitamins, minerals, and trace elements essential for her own health and that of her developing child.

Protein

The word "protein" comes from the greek *proteios,* which means "primary, or holding first place." Since proteins form the basic structure of all living cells and are essential life-forming, life-sustaining elements in human and animal diets, the substance is well named. The building blocks of protein are the amino acids that are yielded upon digestion.

By furnishing amino acids of appropriate numbers and kinds dietary protein promotes the synthesis of specific cellular tissue proteins vital to the growth and maintenance of body tissue. Protein also supplies amino acids for the synthesis of certain enzymes and hormones. Obviously, pregnancy represents a time of intense and highly specialized growth both for the mother and the developing fetus. The American College of Obstetricians and Gynecologists notes that the pregnant woman needs extra protein to provide for the needs of the fetus and to allow for the mother's adjustments due to expanded blood volume and growth of uterine and breast tissue.

Numerous animal studies have been performed in an attempt to discover the effect of protein deprivation on the developing fetus. They have indicated that limiting protein intake in the maternal diet early in pregnancy alters the growth and biochemistry of the brain. However, the smaller the mammal, the more rapid the deterioration of tissues, so restriction of protein in a pregnant rat may be more devastating for the offspring than restriction of protein in a pregnant primate.

One study that bears out this theory involved pregnant monkeys. Monkeys allowed only 50% of optimum protein and/or calorie intake during pregnancy showed only slight changes, suggesting that considerable protein reduction can be made before the brain of the primate fetus is seriously affected. According to D.B. Cheek, editor of *Fetal and Postnatal Cellular Growth*, ". . . the statement that protein restriction per se can cause mental retardation in the human infant would appear to be unproven." However, Cheek warns that severe lack of protein for the entire prenatal period and during infancy, plus poor environment in later years would likely result in brain underdevelopment.

The 1970 and 1973 Conferences of the National Research Council's Committee on Maternal Nutrition raised many questions about the protein requirements of pregnant women. These conferences noted that the pregnant woman's efficient utilization of protein is even lower than had been previously suspected and that protein additions to the diet are therefore highly recommended.

Protein sometimes performs another function, one often overlooked by laymen who think of protein as the body's building blocks and nothing more. In the absence of other available energy sources the body draws energy from dietary protein, thus reducing the amount of amino acids from food protein available for synthesis of body protein. After all, life must be sustained, and energy is required for even the most basic bodily functions. However, this "survival measure" is neither physiologically nor economically desirable. For these reasons a pregnant woman should not only be careful to maintain her protein level at or above the RDA but should also keep carbohydrate and fat intakes at recommended levels. As noted earlier, a severe high-protein, low-carbohydrate diet can bring about tragic consequences. Balance is the important word here, and balance can be achieved by following RDA standards.

Since about 925 grams of protein are deposited during the last six months of pregnancy, RDA calls for an additional 30 grams per day from the second month of pregnancy through delivery. A pregnant woman who adds one pint of milk and two ounces of meat to her regular diet gains these 30 grams. This represents an allowance of 1.3 g of protein per kilogram of body weight for mature women, 1.5 g/kg for pregnant adolescents ages 15 to 18, and 1.7 g/kg for pregnant girls under 15 years of age. This added intake, coupled with adequate energy intake, should be sufficient in most cases. Under these circumstances any protein not needed for growth and tissue development will be used for energy and constitutes no danger to mother or child.

RECOMMENDED DAILY DIETARY ALLOWANCES OF PROTEIN

	Age (years)	Weight (kg)	Weight (lbs)	Height (cm)	Height (ft)	Protein Needs Females (g)	Added During Preg. (g)	Protein Needs Pregnant Females (g)
Non-	11-14	44	97	155	5'2"	44	+30	74
pregnant	15-18	54	119	162	5'5"	48	+30	78
	19-22	58	128	162	5'5"	46	+30	76
	23-50	58	128	162	5'5"	46	+30	76

A look at protein recommendations will threaten the time-honored tradition of giving the largest portion of meat to the adult male. The complete RDA chart reveals that the recommended daily dietary allowance for protein for a 23- to 50-year-old male is 56 g, while a pregnant woman of that same age range should receive 76 g. Protein is food for growth, and the body of a mother-to-be is involved in unique growth processes that require sufficient energy plus sufficient protein.

According to the American College of Obstetricians and Gynecologists, two-thirds of the protein added during pregnancy should be high quality, such as eggs, milk (cheese), and meat. These high-quality foods, all animal in origin, contain the eight essential amino acids that cannot be manufactured by the human body yet are essential to the human adult. The twelve remaining amino acids can be synthesized by the body, provided that enough nitrogen is provided to allow for synthesis.

Other important protein foods (grains, legumes, and nuts) provide the eight essential amino acids only if eaten in certain combinations. Knowing these combinaions is essential if a *vegetarian* diet is to be adequate in protein. The following chart, adapted from the California Department of Public Health Booklet *Nutrition During Pregnancy and Lactation,* shows the combinations needed to ensure against any amino-acid deficiency. For example, grains eaten alone are deficient in two of the eight essential amino acids — isoleucine and lysine. However, certain grains, if combined with certain other vegetable items such as legumes or sesame, provide a diet that no longer lacks these two essential amino acids. Since absence of even one of the eight essential amino acids means that tissue building is impaired, careful study of this chart is essential for any woman who wants to derive protein from nonanimal sources.

The combinations given must be eaten at the same meal in order to constitute a "complete" protein source. Such combinations are easy to make. For example, a whole-wheat-bread and peanut-butter sandwich plus one glass of milk yields a "complete" protein meal. Combination dishes such as green peas and mushrooms or sesame rice are delicious ways of meeting protein needs. If the nonvegetarian serves a meat dish plus these two side dishes, she has provided ample protein, carbohydrates, and several important vitamins and minerals.

COMPLEMENTARY PLANT PROTEIN SOURCES

Food	Amino Acids Deficient	Complementary Protein
Grains	Isoleucine Lysine	Rice + legumes
		Corn + legumes
		Wheat + legumes
		Wheat + peanut + milk
		Wheat + sesame + soybean
		Rice + sesame
		Rice + Brewer's yeast
Legumes	Tryptophan Methionine	Legumes + rice
		Beans + wheat
		Beans + corn
		Soybeans + rice + wheat
		Soybeans + corn + milk
		Soybeans + wheat + sesame
		Soybeans + peanuts + sesame
		Soybeans + peanuts + wheat + rice
		Soybeans + sesame + wheat
Nuts & Seeds	Isoleucine Lysine	Peanuts + sesame + soybeans
		Sesame + beans
		Sesame + soybeans + wheat
		Peanuts + sunflower seeds
Vegetables	Isoleucine	Lima beans, Green peas, Brussel Sprouts, Cauliflower, Broccoli + Sesame seeds or Brazil Nuts or mushrooms
		Greens + millet or converted rice

UNDERSTANDING THE NUTRITIONAL NEEDS OF PREGNANCY — VITAMINS

> With the possible exception of folic acid, there seems to be no scientific justification for prescribing vitamin supplements to healthy pregnant women.
>
> F. E. Hytten and A. M. Thompson
> *(Maternal Nutrition and the Course of Pregnancy*, National Academy of Science, Washington, D. C., 1970)

Energy and protein are vital to the survival and growth of human beings, but energy and protein alone are not enough. Vitamins are also needed to ensure the proper functioning of the body. Near the beginning of this century Casimu Funk, a Polish chemist, discovered what he thought was an amine vital to life. He called that substance "vitamine," or "vital amine," and though the final "e" has since been dropped, the name "vitamin" has come to designate those vital organic substances that are neither carbohydrate, fat, mineral, or protein but are vital to the performance of certain metabolic functions or to the prevention of certain deficiency diseases. Such substances must be supplied in foods, since they cannot be manufactured by the body.

The importance of many fat- and water-soluble vitamins to the developing fetus has been shown in animal laboratory experiments that have produced dietary congenital malformation by withholding Vitamins A, B_{12}, D and E, riboflavin, folic acid, and pantothenic acid from the mother-to-be. However, birth defects occurred only when the mother already had a borderline deficiency herself in the withheld vitamin. Such experiments are delicate, since total omission of vitamins leads to sterility, resorption of the embryo, or stillborn offspring. Severe but not total deprivation leads to malformation of the young. Since humans would rarely duplicate the severe conditions of animal lab experiments, vitamin deficiencies are far less likely to cause abnormalities in human babies. Certainly a slight, temporary lapse below the RDA of a certain vitamin should give no cause for alarm, although prolonged, extreme deprivations could constitute considerable health risk for the mother as well as for the child she carries.

Unfortunately, Americans often consider vitamins as magic elements that can prevent and/or cure sundry ills—if consumed in large enough quantities. Drug manufacturers make a fortune on vitamin preparations, and their advertisements have helped to shift emphasis from vitamin-rich foods to vitamin pills or tonics. Whereas vitamin preparations can and do serve useful purposes in many cases, wholesale consumption of multivitamins or megavitamins is usually a waste of money and can be a dangerous activity. Only in recent years has the public begun to realize that certain vitamins taken in excess are toxic. Since the tablets (both natural and synthetic) are the forms likely to prove toxic, one need not worry that eating too many carrots will cause Vitamin-A toxicity or that eating too many oranges will lead to dangerous Vitamin-C excesses. One should worry, however, about ingesting overdoses of vitamin tablets, especially vitamins A, D, K, C, and B6 (pyridoxine).

In spite of widespread use of vitamin preparations chances are that a person who consumes a well-balanced diet needs no vitamin supplements at all. Even during pregnancy multivitamin preparations are not considered necessary (with the possible exception of folic acid), provided that the mother-to-be is receiving the RDA of all essential vitamins. Since being sure that all vitamins are included in the diet is sometimes difficult, many physicians routinely prescribe multivitamin compounds. Taken as directed, such compounds provide extra insurance against deficiency. Taken in excess, they might well cause complications for the pregnant woman and/or her developing child.

Even when prenatal multivitamins are being taken on a daily basis, a woman's need to eat vitamin-rich foods is not lessened. She should not be misled by the label on her vitamin-pill bottle into thinking that the pill is all that she needs for good health. By eating vitamin-rich foods she is following the most natural method of gaining protection against vitamin deficiency, and at the same time she is gaining calories (energy), minerals, protein, trace elements, and lesser-known vitamins all of which are just as vital to her wellbeing as the vitamins listed on the label of her pill bottle.

The food sources that supply vitamins and the role that each vitamin plays in bodily functions should be well understood by any expectant mother who wishes to provide the ideal nutritional environment for the growth and development of her child. The following chart provides this information in capsule form — no pun intended!

Vitamins are usually divided into two broad groups—fat soluble (A, D, E, K) and water-soluble (C and B-complex).

A discussion of the reasons that pregnancy may increase the need for certain fat-soluble vitamins follows the charts below.

RECOMMENDED DIETARY ALLOWANCES OF FAT-SOLUBLE VITAMINS

Fat-soluble Vitamins

	Age (years)	Weight (kg)	Weight (lbs)	Height (cm)	Height (ft)	Vitamin A Activity (RE)*	Vitamin A Activity (IU)	Vitamin D (IU)	Vitamin E Activity (IU)
Non-	11-14	44	97	155	5'2"	800	4,000	400	12
pregnant	15-18	54	119	162	5'5"	800	4,000	400	12
	19-22	58	128	162	5'5"	800	4,000	400	12
	23-50	58	128	162	5'5"	800	4,000		12
Pregnant						1000	5,000	400	15

*Retinol equiv.

A pregnant woman should include 1000 RE (5000 IU) of vitamin A in her daily diet during the last half of pregnancy. This 20% increase is believed necessary for optimum cell development, tooth formation, normal bone growth, vision, and maintenance of integrity of epithelial tissue. This amount also allows for storage of vitamin A by the fetus.

FAT SOLUBLE VITAMINS — OVERVIEW

Vitamin	Dietary Sources	Bodily Functions	Deficiency Symptoms
A	Liver, red meats, cream, butter, whole milk, egg yolk, fortified margarine, green and yellow vegetables, yellow fruits	Maintenance of epithelial tissue; essential to production of visual pigment; promotes growth, reproduction, other metabolic processes	Night blindness, xerophthalmia, skin and mucous membrane infections
D	Fortified milk and margarine, eggs, fish oils	Increases calcium and phosphorous absorption, promotes mineralization and growth of bones	Rickets, osteomalacia
E	Vegetable oils, nuts, eggs, milk, fish, leafy vegetables, dried green split peas, whole grains, wheat germ	Antioxidant; protects red blood cells	Possibly anemia
K	Cheese, egg yolk, liver, green, leafy vegetables	Aids in blood clotting	Hemorrhagic disease of newborn

Since synthetic vitamin A can be toxic in significant overdoses, it should be taken only under a doctor's supervision. Twenty to thirty times the RDA of this vitamin can cause anorexia (loss of appetite), hyperirritability, skin lesions, bone decalcification, and headaches. For infants from one to three months of age doses as low as 18,500 IU of water-dispersed Vitamin A and D (approximately the number of IUs in the standard 50 ml bottle of infant A-and-D vitamins) can be toxic. In light of these facts the mother-to-be who routinely ingests large amounts of synthetic Vitamin A may well be endangering her own health and that of her child.

Adequate exposure to sunlight means adequate production of vitamin D, but in cold climates or other situations where adequate exposure to sunlight is difficult, vitamin-D deficiency can result. For this reason many foods, notably milk, are vitamin-D fortified. Since fortification has become widespread in the United States, rickets due to vitamin-D deficiency is extremely rare beyond infancy. Beyond age 22 no RDA has been set for nonpregnant females, provided adequate exposure to sunlight is possible.

Although the pregnant female may be exposed to sunlight and may be drinking large amounts of Vitamin-D-fortified milk, the National Research Council has still recommended the daily inclusion of 400 IU. The increased need for calcium and phosphorus by fetal skeletal tissue calls for more than the usual amounts of vitamin D to promote absorption and utilization of these two minerals. Provided that the recommended 400 IUs of vitamin D are obtained in vitamin-rich foods such as egg yolk, liver, fortified milk, butter, and margarine, the pregnant woman does not need to think of supplementation. The pregnant *vegetarian* who does not include fortified milk or other such foods in her diet may be subject to Vitamin-D deficiency and should discuss possible supplementation with her doctor. If a supplement is used, care should be taken to avoid overdosing. Excessive amounts of this vitamin (1000—3000 IU/kg/day) are dangerous to both children and adults. Vitamin D facilitates absorption of calcium, and hypercalcemia (fever, muscular weakness, loss of appetite, nausea, excessive thirst, constipation) in infants and children has been linked to vitamin-D intoxication. Kidney disorders in children and adults have been traced to overdoses of vitamin D. When English health authorities overfortified milk with this vitamin, a severe outbreak of mental disorders occurred. Occasional vitamin-D sensitivity results in adverse affects even if intake is relatively low. In view of the many foods now fortified with vitamin D many persons may already be receiving daily dietary amounts larger than the 400 IU set by the National Research Council.

Since no known benefits result from excessive doses and since evidence suggests that such overdoses may be harmful, supplementation should be considered only if no food sources of the vitamin are available. If supplementation does seem necessary, it should be limited to no more than the recommended 400 IU per day. The pregnant woman should be especially careful to avoid taking too much vitamin D. Recent studies suggest that, in cases in which the mother is sensitive to this vitamin, excessive intakes may be a significant cause of mental retardation in the offspring. Though this relationship has not yet been proven in humans, a mother-to-be should not risk large intakes.

As pregnant women increase their calorie level, they should be sure that additional vitamin E (a total of 15 IU) is included in the diet in order to make up for the amount desposited in the fetus. Placental transfer of vitamin E is relatively poor, and the infant probably gets only enough of the vitamin to meet his immediate needs.

No toxicity symptoms have been noted, even at daily levels as high as 800

RECOMMENDED DAILY DIETARY ALLOWANCES OF WATER-SOLUBLE VITAMINS

	Non-pregnant Women				Pregnant Women
Age (years)	11-14	15-18	19-22	23-50	
Weight (g)	44	54	58	58	
Weight (pounds)	97	119	128	128	
Height (cm)	155	162	162	162	
Height (feet)	5'2"	5'5"	5'5"	5'5"	
Vitamin					
C (Ascorbic Acid) (mg)	45	45	45	45	60
B_9 (Folacin or Folic Acid) (mg)	0.4	0.4	0.4	0.4	0.8
B_5 (Niacin or Nictonic Acid) (mg)	16	14	14	13	+2
B_2 (Riboflavin) (mg)	1.3	1.4	1.4	1.2	+0.3
B_1 (Thiamin) (mg)	1.2	1.1	1.1	1.0	+0.3
B_6 (Pyridoxine) (mg)	1.6	2.0	2.0	2.0	2.5
B_{12} (Cobalamin) (mg)	.003	.003	.003	.003	.004

IU/kg of body weight ingested for up to five months. However, there is recent evidence that overdoses of vitamin E block the effectiveness of vitamin K and produce excessive bleeding similar to that seen in vitamin-K-deficiency cases. Since there is no proof that excessive amounts accomplish the health miracles that many claim for this vitamin, pregnant women would do well to avoid taking megadoses of vitamin E.

Since under normal conditions the intestinal tract synthesizes enough vitamin K to meet the body's needs, the pregnant woman is not advised to take vitamin K supplements. In fact, excessive doses of one form of that vitamin have been known to produce hemolytic anemia in rats and kernicterus (a potential cause of brain damage) in premature human infants. Recent studies have indicated that administration of large doses of one form of vitamin K to a pregnant woman shortly before delivery is potentially dangerous to the unborn child. For this reason pregnant females are not allowed any over-the-counter supplements of that particular form of the vitamin, though they may be allowed to use Vitamin K_1.

Since there is no proven reason for ingesting synthetic vitamin K except in extreme cases and there is evidence as to the vitamin's potential harmful effects, a pregnant woman should avoid synthetic preparations unless prescribed by her physician. Fortunately, in its natural form Vitamin K does not have these adverse affects, so there is no need to worry about consuming too many foods rich in the vitamin.

The following overview gives RDA requirements of water-soluble vitamins for non-pregnant and pregnant women.

For the non-pregnant female 45 mg of vitamin C daily is considered adequate, though in the presence of fevers and infections, severe burns, or major surgery, a physician may recommend greater amounts. For the pregnant woman 60 mg daily is recommended, approximately the amount found in four ounces of orange juice.

Recent research by Linus Pauling has indicated that large doses (from 0.5 to 5 g per day) of vitamin C may reduce the frequency and severity of the common cold, but any such benefits would not be considered nutritional functions of the vitamin. Since such claims aren't well substantiated, consumption of excessive amounts is not recommended, unless such amounts are ordered by a physician. Even then a pregnant woman might wish to deliberate before consuming large quantities of the vitamin. Prenatal overdosing with vitamin C (synthetic, megavitamin form) can raise the daily level well over 400 mg, possibly predisposing the child to vitamin-C deficiency. In this way a child may be conditioned to need amounts far beyond the normal ones. In view of this potential danger pregnant women would do well to avoid overdosing with vitamin C in its synthetic form.

As in the case of Vitamin C, the B-complex vitamins were discovered through man's search for the cause of a widespread disease. This disease, beriberi, caused many deaths before it was related to the lack of a vitamin element that was first called water-soluble B. As that element came to be better understood, scientists discovered that an entire complex of vitamins had been placed under that umbrella designation. Subsequent research led to the isolation of the various B-complex vitamins and verification of some of the important functions of each.

WATER-SOLUBLE-VITAMIN OVERVIEW

Vitamin	Dietary Sources	Bodily Functions	Deficiency Symptoms
C (Ascorbic Acid)	Citrus fruits, tomatoes, cabbage, green peppers, strawberries, cantaloupes	Aids in iron absorption; cements body cells together; strengthens gums	Scurvy, slow wound healing, epithelial hemorrhages
B_9 (Folacin or Folic Acid)	Legumes, green vegetables, whole wheat products, asparagus, liver, kidney, heart	Amino acid metabolism	Gastrointestinal disturbances, diarrhea, red tongue, sprue, mega blastic anemia
B_5 (Niacin or Nicotnic Acid)	Liver, meats, yeast, dried beans and peas, whole-grain cereals	Aids in utilization of fats and proteins; aids in energy metabolism	Pellagra, dermatitis, neuritis
B_2 (Ribo-flavin)	Milk, liver, enriched cereals, cheese, eggs, leafy vegetables	Energy metabolism	Reddened lips, cracks at corners of mouth, eye irritation
B_1 (Thiamin)	Pork, milk, lima beans, dried beans and peas, wheat germ, whole-grain and enriched breads, whole-grain and enriched cereals, leafy and green vegetables	Aids in carbohydrate utilization	Beriberi, gastrointestinal disorders, loss of eye coordination
B_6 (Pyri-doxine)	Wheat, corn, meat, nuts, liver, yeast, fish, dried green split peas, whole-grain cereals, green, leafy vegetables	Aids in synthesis and utilization of amino acids	Anemia, kidney stones, central-nervous-system abnormalities (convulsions, irritability, muscular twitching), dermatitis
B_{12} (Coba-lamin)	Liver, kidney, milk, muscle meats, fish, eggs, cheese (not present in plant foods)	Constituent of bone marrow, helps form red blood cells; protein synthesis	Pernicious anemia, sprue, neurological disorders

The increased metabolic rate of pregnancy, with the accompanying need for increased caloric intake, means that more thiamin is needed (vitamin B_1). By adding 0.3 mg of vitamin B_1 to her recommended nonpregnant level an expectant mother can prevent thiamin deficiency. Recent findings indicate that the need for thiamin is greatest during the final three months of gestation.

Based on a recommended dietary allowance of 0.6 mg per 1,000 kcal, the riboflavin needs of nonpregnant women reflect the growth and developmental requirements evident in their recommended caloric intakes. Due to increased energy requirements pregnant women should add 0.3 mg per day of riboflavin, or vitamin B_2, to the RDA for their age group. The pregnant vegetarian who does not use milk should be sure to include plenty of legumes, whole grains, and enriched breads and cereals in her diet to offset the possibility of deficiency in vitamin B2, or riboflavin.

As the chart indicates, the RDA for niacin or vitamin B5, is based on caloric intake, with 6.6 mg per 1,000 kcal recommended for adults and not less than 13 mg at caloric levels less than 2,000. Though the niacin needs of the pregnant woman are not clearly understood, a daily increase of 2 mg of niacin above the nonpregnant RDA is advised in line with the recommended increase of 300 kcal per day.

Recommended daily dietary allowances for pyridoxine, or vitamin B6, for nonpregnant young females has been set at 1.6, while for older women the RDA is 2.0. Since recent studies have indicated that women using oral contraceptives may require B6 in amounts far greater than the supply available in the average diet, physicians sometimes administer supplemental B6. However, doses must be at least 10 times greater than RDA in order to be effective. Since excessive amounts of B6 have been known to interfere with protein metabolism, such high intakes of vitamin B6 may be ill-advised.

Pregnant women need at least 2.5 mg of vitamin B6 per day. Placental blood shows as much as five times the amount of B6 as mother's blood, an indication that the fetus is being given a store of this important vitamin. Occasionally, certain biochemical abnormalities of pregnant women on "normal" diets have been corrected through use of pyridoxine administrations. This may indicate that even higher levels of B6 are needed during pregnancy. Hyperemesis (severe morning sickness with excessive vomiting) has been treated by administering vitamin B6, but there is no proof that the practice is warranted.

In view of the fact that B6 dependency has been induced in normal human adults after 33 days of 20-mg doses of pyridoxine, a pregnant woman should not experiment on her own with megadoses of this vitamin. In one instance a mother who received injections of vitamin B6 during pregnancy gave birth to an infant who developed seizures controllable only by use of pyridoxine hydrochloride. This case and others suggesting the possibility of inducing B6 dependence by prenatal use of the drug seem to outweight any possible advantages of self-prescribed superdosing with pyridoxine.

Recommended daily dietary allowance of folacin, or vitamin B9, for nonpregnant women has normally been set at 0.4 mg, an amount that should prevent deficiency symptoms except in extreme cases. Unusual circumstances, including excessive consumption of alcohol, sometimes increase the body's folic-acid demands. For pregnant women that allowance is doubled, for many studies have indicated that folic-acid requirements are greatly increased during pregnancy. A 1967 study ascribing fetal damage to folic-acid deficiency has led scientists to raise B9 allowances for the protection of the fetus and for preservation of the mother's own stores. The American College of Obstetricians and Gynecologists has recommended 0.4 to 0.8 mg supplementary doses of folic acid as insurance against damage to the fetus, and many authorities agree that supplementation is wise, though they differ as to the number of miligrams per day. Patients with low hemoglobin levels and those with multiple fetuses may need unusually high levels of folic acid, but a physician should prescribe any supplementation beyond 0.8 mg per day.

Since Cobalamin,or vitamin B12, is relatively abundant in animal foods, natural dietary deficiencies are most likely to occur in true vegetarians who avoid milk and eggs as well as meat.

Supplementation is recommended for strict *vegetarians*, since they may develop sour tongue, paresthesias (burning, tingling skin), amenorrhea (abnormal absence of mestruation), low serum-B12 levels, and degeneration of the spinal cord, even if they show no signs of anemia. Vegetarians who ingest large amounts of folic acid, masking any signs of pernicious anemia, are particularly susceptible to serious neurological damage. The lacto-ovo vegetarian who receives at least four glasses of cow's milk daily is not in danger of B12 deficiency, but soybean and goat's milk do not contain sufficient amounts of B12, and lacto-ovo vegetarians who use these milks exclusively may require supplementation. Pregnant women should increase their B12 intake to 4 ug (0.004 mg) daily to compensate for the B12 demands of the fetus.

Other B-complex vitamins may later be placed on the RDA chart, but at this time no deficiency seems likely to occur under normal circumstances, so no recommended daily dietary allowances have yet been set for the vitamins pantothenic acid, lipoic acid, and biotin and for the pseudovitamins paraaminobenzoic acid, inositol, and choline. Since no conclusive data exists to indicate that pregnancy increases demands for these substances and since large supplements might prove dangerous to the health of mother or child, a pregnant woman should avoid any such supplements unless they are prescribed by her physician to combat a particular disorder.

UNDERSTANDING THE NUTRITIONAL NEEDS OF PREGNANCY— MINERALS AND TRACE ELEMENTS

> It is difficult to justify limitation of table salt in healthy women during pregnancy on the basis of either animal or clinical evidence.
>
> Committee on Dietary Allowances,
> Food and Nutrition Board, National Research
> Council *(Recommended Dietary Allowances,*
> 8th edition, National Academy of Sciences,
> Washington, D. C., 1974)

Minerals in nature seem inert and lifeless, yet within the human body they are active, performing life-sustaining functions as regulators, transmitters, controllers, activators, and builders. The National Research Council's Committee on Dietary Allowances has divided minerals into two groups, those needed in levels of 100 mg per day or more and those needed in amounts no greater than a few mg per day. In keeping with this distinction minerals will be grouped according to this format.

For the pregnant woman maintaining sufficient calcium intake is vitally important, since this element is essential to such a large number of life-sustaining processes, many of which are greatly taxed by pregnancy. The rapid mineralization of fetal skeletal tissue during the last half of gestation requires enough additional calcium to call for a 50% increase in recommended daily dietary allowances for pregnant women, thus raising their RDA to 1,200 mg per day. If maternal calcium intake has previously been adequate, prenatal intakes of 1,200 mg are sufficient for both mother and child. If the mother's intake has not been adequate, the fetus tends to use calcium from maternal stores, causing demineralization of the mother's bones. In severe deprivation cases the mother might experience irreversible bone damage. The pregnant vegetarian who avoids milk and other dairy products should realize that under most circumstances only about 300 mg of calcium per day are supplied by nondairy sources, and this falls far below the 1,200 mg per day recommended during pregnancy

MINERALS AND TRACE ELEMENTS

Group I	Group II (Trace Elements)	
Calcium	Iron	
Phosphorus	Iodine	Manganese
Magnesium	Zinc	Molybdenum
Sodium	Fluoride	Selenium
Chloride	Copper	Chromium
Potassium	Cobalt	

RECOMMENDED DAILY DIETARY ALLOWANCES OF MINERALS

	Non-pregnant Women				Pregnant Women
Age (years)	11-14	15-18	19-22	23-50	
Weight (g)	44	54	58	58	
Weight (pounds)	97	119	128	128	
Height (cm)	155	162	162	162	
Height (feet)	5'2"	5'5"	5'5"	5'5"	
Mineral					
Calcium (mg)	1200	1200	800	800	1200
Phosphorus (mg)	1200	1200	800	800	1200
Iodine (mg)	.115	.115	.100	.100	.125
Iron (mg)	18	18	18	18	36
Magnesium (mg)	300	300	300	300	450
Zinc (mg)	15	15	15	15	20

Note: Supplementary iron needs for pregnant women cannot be met by ordinary diets. Mineral absorption is inhibited by excessive use of antacids. Even if RDA standards are met for each of the minerals listed above, frequent use of antacids can lead to mineral-deficiency symptoms. Especially during pregnancy a woman should seek other means of preventing or relieving acid indigestion.

by the National Research Council. Calcium tablets can be prescribed for a no-milk vegetarian, but calcium derived from milk is still preferable. The lactose in milk plus the vitamin D in fortified milk apparently increase calcium absorption.

As noted earlier, no clinical evidence of calcium toxicity exists, though reports have linked leg cramps in late pregnancy to possible imbalance in the serum calcium-to-phosphorus ratio and to the fairly high phosphorus content of milk. To exclude milk from the prenatal diet in hopes of lessening leg cramps is ill-advised, since calcium need is at its highest during the final trimester of pregnancy.

Phosphorus recommended daily dietary allowances are equal to those of calcium, with 1,200 mg of phosphorus recommended for nonpregnant females 11 to 18 years of age and 800 mg for nonpregnant females over 18 years of age. Since phosphorus demands seem to be greater during pregnancy, allowances are raised to 1,200 mg per day during the prenatal period.

Recommended daily dietary allowance of magnesium for non-pregnant women has been set at 300 mg per day, with an increase of 150 mg (total of 450 mg) advised for pregnant women. Although large oral intakes do not seem harmful to persons with normal kidney function, doses as high as 3 to 5 g (3,500 to 5,000 mg) have a cathartic or laxative effect that may make excessive prenatal intakes ill-advised.

Though no recommended daily dietary allowance for sodium appears on the National Research Council's chart, any discussion of prenatal dietary needs should include information on sodium and chloride intakes. Like the word "calorie," the term "sodium" has had primarily negative connotations for most pregnant women. Warnings to "cut down on salt" or "hide that salt shaker" have made many women assume that salt (sodium chloride) is too dangerous to be allowed in their daily diets. Before considering the reasons why such fears have become part of general pregnancy lore, a look at the separate functions of the two components of table salt, sodium and chloride, should enable one to see dietary salt in a more positive light.

Sodium, the principal cation (positive ion) of extracellular fluid, helps to maintain the body's fluid balance and acid-base balance. Along with potassium, the principal cation of intracellular fluid, sodium controls such vital functions as cellular excitability and nerve-impulse conduction. Animal studies have shown that a deficiency of either cation results in growth retardation. One nutritionist has pointed out that "Perhaps no other physiologic activity is so broad in scope or so profound in its effect on body symptoms (especially the cardiovascular, renal and gastrointestinal systems) as the mechanisms by which the fluid-electrolyte and acid-base balances are maintained." Essential to life itself, these delicate mechanisms are partially controlled by sodium.

MINERALS OVERVIEW

Mineral	Dietary Source	Bodily Functions	Deficiency Symptoms
Calcium	Milk, cheese, dark green vegetables, dried legumes	Tooth and bone formation, blood clotting, nerve transmission, muscle contraction and relaxation, heart action	Rickets, stunted growth, osteoporosis, convulsions, tetany
Phosphorus	Milk, cheese, meat, egg yolk; whole grains, legumes, nuts, poultry	Bone and tooth formation, acid-base balance, overall metabolism, buffer system	Sprue, celiac disease, tetany, demineralization of bone, loss of calcium
Iodine	Marine fish, shellfish, iodized salt	Synthesis of thyroid hormone that regulates cell oxidation	Endemic colloid goiter, endemic cretinism
Iron	Liver, meats, egg yolks, whole grains, dark green vegetables, legumes, nuts, enriched bread and cereal, molasses, dried fruits	Hemoglobin formation, cellular oxidation	Anemia, weakness, reduced resistance to infection
Magnesium	Whole grains, nuts, milk, meat, legumes, green, leafy vegetables	Constituent of bones and teeth, coenzyme in carbohydrate and protein metabolism,	Growth failure, behaviorial disturbances, weakness, spasms muscle and nerve irritability
Zinc	Liver, seafood	Essential enzyme constituent	Growth failure, small sex glands

Complete restriction of salt means lowering chloride as well as sodium levels. The most important anion (negative ion) in the maintenance of fluid and electrolyte balance, chloride is also vital to the formation of hydrochloric acid, essential to the formation of human digestive fluids. Since chloride is a chief component of these gastric juices, severe, prolonged vomiting or diarrhea may cause significant losses that may call for supplementation. Severe chloride losses of this type may lead to disturbances in the body's acid-base metabolism, notably hypochloremic alkaosis, a condition characterized by irritability or, in severe cases, normocalcemic tetany.

Since table salt is almost the sole source of chloride, persons on strict salt-restriction regimens may require an alternative chloride source to ensure against disturbance of digestive activity or acid-base and fluid-electroltye balances. Any supplementation should, of course, be undertaken only under a physician's orders.

If sodium and chloride are essential to life, why has sodium-chloride restriction become almost routine dietary advice for pregnant women? When latest National Research Council reports indicate that pregnancy *increases* the body's sodium requirements by a total of 25 g over nine months, or approximately 92 mg per day, why are some doctors still advising total restriction of table salt for certain patients? When severe vomiting in early pregnancy makes chloride deficiency a serious possibility for some women, why increase the likelihood of such deficiency by outlawing all dietary sodium chloride?

To understand the reasons why salt has so often been restricted in prenatal diets, one must recall the earlier discussion of toxemia, "the disease of theories." Edema (fluid retention) is one of the symptoms of toxemia, and that symptom has long been treated by limiting salt intake and/or administering diuretics. In fact, the 1975 edition of one handbook that is currently widely distributed by the country's obstetricians states, "If even one of the symptoms [of toxemia] is present, salt intake must be reduced or eliminated." Such written advice tempts many women to do their own prescribing, and they may eliminate salt without consulting their doctors, who might now differ with the handbook.

However, such advice is still routinely given by many physicians in spite of the fact that *Nutrition in Maternal Health Care,* a pamphlet published in 1974 by the American College of Obstretricians and Gynecologists, has noted: "Sodium is required in pregnancy for the expanded maternal tissue and fluid compartments as well as to provide for fetal needs. Concepts of sodium metabolism in pregnancy appear to be in the process of change. The older and more traditional view is that of an insidious retainer in which sodium is apt to increase vascular reactivity and predispose to toxemia. This is being challenged by a more current theory that if adequate sodium intake is not maintained, the pregnant woman can go into shock. Which of these two opposing views is correct cannot be ascertained at present. From a clinical point of view, however, it appears reasonable to permit the normal patient to use the level of sodium intake she prefers."

The members of the National Research Council's Committee on Dietary Allowances reached a similar conclusion. Indeed, in recent animal experiments undesirable effects have been noted when pregnant rats are sodium-restricted. Citing this and other studies, the National Research Council's Food and Nutrition Board advises against routine restrictions of sodium chloride from prenatal diets and also against the often concurrent practice of administering diuretics, noting that "the routine use of diuretics without specific clinical indications is unwise."

In view of the conflicting views on the subject what should a pregnant woman do about salt restriction? First, she should definitely *not* severely limit her salt intake of her own accord, all advice from well-meaning friends and relatives notwithstanding. Avoiding overuse of salt by not adding salt to foods that she has seasoned during cooking is probably one safe way to keep sodium-chloride intake at desirable levels. She should not begin exclusive use of new potassium-chloride salt substitutes without first checking with her doctor. Secondly, she should resist the temptation to use self-prescribed diuretics as a means of cheating on weight checkups. Such tampering with weight by sudden loss of body fluids not only gives the physician a false picture of the progress of pregnancy but also may result in excessive losses of sodium. Thirdly, if she is routinely advised to exclude all sodium chloride from her prenatal diet, she may feel justified in questioning that opinion, citing the latest recommendation of the American College of Obstetricians and Gynecologists and the National Research Council's Committee on Recommended Dietary Allowances. She might wish to provide her physician with quotations from these two sources. Finally, if complications such as hypertension (high blood pressure) make sodium restriction necessary, she should make every effort to follow her physician's orders concerning use of table salt. In addition, if she reduces the amount of ham, bacon, chips, and other high-salt or high-sodium-benzoate foods in her diet, she can reduce sodium intake still further. However, in cases of drastic reduction in salt intake she might ask her physician's opinion as to the wisdom of using a chloride supplement, at least for the duration of pregnancy.

One further point should be mentioned concerning restricted salt intake. As the section on iodine shows, iodized salt is a prime source of iodine, a mineral essential to the prevention of endemic goiter *and* endemic cretinism. Mild iodine supplementation may be necessary for a woman who must eliminate salt from her diet due to hypertension or other medical problems. Under certain conditions failure to receive such supplementation may mean potential tragedy for the pregnant woman, especially if she lives in the "goiter belt" of the United States. Conversely, large self-prescribed iodine supplements might have undesirable side effects. Any tablet supplementation should therefore be undertaken only under a doctor's supervision and *only* if a woman falls into a high-risk iodine-deficiency group. As current studies of iodine intakes show that increasingly fewer women fall into high-risk groups, a pregnant woman should seek the latest possible data on iodine before agreeing to supplementary doses of this mineral.

As noted above, potassium is the body's major cation (positively charged ion) of intracellular fluid and is vital to the maintenance of acid-base and fluid-electrolyte balance, muscle activity, carbohydrate activity, and protein synthesis. Since potassium is widely distributed in common foods, potassium deficiency due solely to insufficient intakes is extremely rare. Deficiency due to excessive loss of potassium through severe diarrhea and/or vomiting or prolonged use of certain diuretics does occur and may require potassium supplementation to prevent serious complications. Since no deficiency is likely except under such special circumstances, no recommended daily dietary allowance has been set. The average American diet includes from 2 to 4 mg per day, an amount assumed to be adequate for pregnant as well as nonpregnant women.

Of the 17 trace elements for which biological functions in animals have been demonstrated only 10 have been evaluated in terms of human nutrition and only 3 of these (iron, iodine, and zinc) appear on the RDA charts, though fluoride levels are given within the general text of the 1974 edition and are therefore discussed in this guide.

In view of the complexity of the iron-absorption process, the best way to ensure adequate intake of iron is to maintain a well-balanced diet that includes the recommended daily dietary allowance of iron. While that allowance is one that the average male can meet by diet alone, females may not be able to meet iron RDA without supplementation.

Throughout her active reproduction years a woman needs 18 mg of iron per day, enough to offset the loss of iron due to menstruation. Two-thirds of menstruating women are unable to accumulate adequate stores of iron, since they deplete their stores during each menstrual period. Though anemia may not develop in nonpregnant women, the average American woman loses iron at the rate of 0.5 mg per day during her menstrual period, and 5% of normal women experience losses as high as 1.4 mg per day. With monthly losses of this magnitude it is easy to see why iron stores are rarely sufficient to meet the stresses of pregnancy. Iron intakes of 18 mg per day for the nonpregnant woman would allow iron stores to be maintained, stores that could be utilized under the stress imposed by pregnancy. If this RDA is met throughout the child-bearing years, menstrual losses can be replenished and tissue and liver reserves restored after each pregnancy.

Unfortunately, most American women who enter pregnancy have not followed an 18-mg-per-day iron regimen for most of their lives. Many are already borderline anemics, and others quickly become anemic as pregnancy progresses. To offset the possibility of anemia, the National Research Council has recommended that mothers-to-be not only upgrade their dietary iron supplies but also take iron supplements, especially during the last half of pregnancy.

Iron is an essential element of hemoglobin, and with a 20% to 40% increase in maternal circulating blood, a mother-to-be needs a good supply of the building blocks of hemoglobin. If her pre-pregnancy iron stores were low or nonexistent, she may rapidly approach an anemic state even during the first few months of pregnancy. If she has a past history of anemia, her chances of becoming anemic again are greatly increased by pregnancy.

An estimated 6 mg of iron per day are needed for the manufacture of maternal blood cells and for the growth of the fetus. This iron may be partially obtained from maternal iron stores, though the average healthy American woman has only 0.3 g of iron in reserve, and these stores alone would barely provide enough iron for the first two months of pregnancy. Once these stores are depleted, the hemoglobic level of the blood falls rapidly, and anemia is soon diagnosed.

Of course, maternal stores are not the body's only means of meeting the iron demands of pregnancy. An iron-rich prenatal diet can help to supply this vital mineral, yet even the most conscientious mother-to-be will find it difficult to ingest enough iron to ensure the absorption of the necessary 6 to 7 mg per day, since only 10% to 12% of food iron is likely to be absorbed and utilized by the body. For example; the average American prenatal diet contains 12 to 15 mg of iron, of which only about 12% (3.0 mg) is utilized, leaving a deficit of 3 to 4 mg. That deficit can best be met by the use of a ferrous-iron supplement. The National Research Council recommends that all pregnant women receive 30 to 60 mg of iron per day during the second and third trimesters of pregnancy, since absorption of 20% of that amount would ensure sufficient iron to meet the demands of pregnancy without depleting the mother's stores and/or leading to anemia. No deficiency is likely at these levels, nor is iron overload.

The American College of Obstetricians and Gynecologists, recognizing the fact that most women are unable to meet the needs of pregnancy by iron stores alone or even by iron stores plus an iron-rich diet, has recommended supplemental iron as soluble ferrous salts in amounts of 30 to 60 mg per day during pregnancy and for two or three months afterward (to replace maternal stores). Since a well-balanced diet would not likely contain such high concentrations of iron, a pregnant woman should seriously consider the use of an iron supplement in the amounts recommended by the National Research Council and the American College of Obstetricians and Gynecologists.

Most persons do not consume adequate amounts of seafood and/or iodine-rich eggs and dairy products to meet the body's requirements for iodine, routine use of iodized salt is currently recommended.

Since iodized salt currently provides .76 mg of iodine per gram and since the average person consumes about 3.4 g of salt per day, use of iodized salt should enable a woman to meet the RDA for iodine. Unfortunately, iodized salt makes up only slightly more than half of the table salt consumed in the United States. This is partly due to the fact that most salt bought in bulk quantities has not been iodine-enriched, making it unlikely that preprocessed foods or foods cooked in restaurants and schools contain it.

Health-food enthusiasts currently using sea salt should realize that such salt is not iodized, despite the fact that it comes from the sea, the home of iodine-rich seafood. Women would be well-advised to use iodized salt in all home food preparation, since this may be the only chance to be sure that the family's RDA for iodine is met.

Since excessive intakes of iodine have been known to block the production of thyroid hormone and cause goiter and other complications, megadoses are not recommended. Vegetarians who include unusually large amounts of kelp and cabbage in their diets should realize that these goitrogens (goiter producers if used in excessive amounts) may also block thyroid-hormone production. Pregnant women and young girls at the puberty stage form the highest risk group for development of endemic goiter (goitor due to iodine deficiency). The increased demands of the fetus drain the mother's own stores, thus leaving her vulnerable to goiter development.

Unfortunately, iodine deficiency during pregnancy presents far more serious problems than the development of endemic goiter. Cretinism has been linked to a deficiency of thyroid hormone during the fetal period, a deficiency that might be traced to iodine deficiency in the prenatal diet. As early as 1871 C.G. Flagge, an English doctor, noted that "Goiter is the earlier effect of the endemic influence; cretinism shows itself when the action of that influence is intesified by operating on more than one generation." Characterized by dwarfism, sparse hair, distended abdomen (pot belly), puffy eyes, enlarged tongue, thickened lips, depressed nose bridge, and dry, thickened, yellowish skin, this syndrome is seen most often in the Middle East. Relatively rare in America, it is often not recognized until about the third month. From this time on chronic constipation, increased lethargy, inability to sit up, and signs of mental retardation may appear. Parents may believe that the infant's symptoms indicate mongolism, but a physician can usually distinguish between the two conditions even at birth. Though early treatment with thyroid hormone has proven successful in improving physical growth of the congenital cretin, some degree of mental retardation is very likely to persist in spite of treatment.

To offset the increased possibility of iodine deficiency and its resultant problems for both mother and child, the National Research Council has set recommended daily allowances of iodine for pregnant women at .125 mg. For many women use of iodized salt is essential if this RDA is to be met. Compounding the difficulties already described concerning intake of sufficient amounts of iodized salt to meet recommended daily allowances is the "cut out the salt" edict so often issued to the pregnant woman at the slightest sign of water retention.With endemic goiter and endemic cretinism as potential results of an iodine-deficient prenatal diet, the routine restriction of table salt for pregnant women is again called into question. For those relatively few women who fall into the high-risk iodine-deficiency category a dietary restriction imposed because it might possibly prevent toxemia could lead to iodine deficiency severe enough to cause endemic cretinism. If severe salt restriction is seen as absolutely necessary, such high-risk women might need a physician's help in meeting iodine needs.

As insurance against deficiency symptoms the National Research Council has set RDA for zinc at 15 mg per day for nonpregnant women, with an additional 5 mg per day for pregnant women.The importance of adequate zinc intakes to a pregnant woman is evident if one notes that even transient zinc deficiencies during the intrauterine state can have permanent effects in animals. This fact should not lead mothers-to-be to ingest large zinc supplements, for such supplements should be used only under a doctor's supervision and only if there is clear evidence of zinc deficiency.

Though it is not listed on the RDA chart, fluoride is discussed within the text of the RDA manual as an element incorporated in the structure of teeth and bones. Recognized as an essential element for resistance to tooth decay, fluoride is assumed to be abundant enough in soils, water supplies, and plant and animal foods so that no recommended daily dietary allowance has been set.

Besides its known role in the prevention of tooth decay fluoride is now being cited as an agent essential to overall physical growth and development and to the prevention of osteoporosis (soft bones of elderly people) and Paget's disease (a disease of bone metabolism). Especially because of its proven effectiveness in prevention of dental caries fluoride has been added to many water supplies across the country. At the current additive rate of 1 ppm there is no danger of toxicity. Many indications of lowered incidence of tooth decay will probably mean that fluoridation of water supplies will become more and more commonplace.

Excess fluoride can produce endemic dental fluorosis (mottling or discoloration of tooth enamel), but such excessive amounts are normally observed only in communities where *natural* fluoride content of the water supply is unusually high. Teeth of babies in these high-fluoride areas are affected by fluoride excesses (greater than 2ppm) in the budding stage, so that they are mottled, discolored, and pitted when they appear. Such teeth do have unusually high resistance to cavities, but their mottled appearance is a high price to pay for no dental caries. Even more serious than mottling of teeth is osteosclerosis, or abnormal density of the skeletal bone, a condition that can cause crippling. Occurring in adults who habitually ingest excessive amounts of fluoride, this disorder would not be likely to exist in areas with no *natural* high-fluoride problems.

For pregnant and nonpregnant women alike fluoride is an essential element. Women who ingest fluoridated drinking water at 1ppm are highly unlikely to have any deficiency problems, and even those who do not live in communities with fluoridation programs will probably get sufficient amounts of this element from water that is naturally high in fluoride. Though a person would need to ingest from 20 to 80 mg per day over a period of many years to produce a toxic effect, there seems to be no evidence to warrant any supplementation program beyond the 1ppm currently added to water supplies. Taking large doses would be ill-advised during the prenatal period, except under unusual circumstances or if additional supplementation is prescribed by a physician.

About the remaining trace elements known to be essential to human health there is too little information to allow RDAs to be set. Fortunately, deficiencies of these trace elements are unlikely to occur in women on well-balanced diets that include a minimum of highly refined and processed foods.

For example, copper, essential for prevention of anemia, skeletal defects, degeneration of the nervous system, reproductive failure and other serious disorders, is abundant in such foods as liver, kidney, shellfish, nuts, dried legumes, and raisins. Copper deficiency, extremely rare in man, is usually seen when other disorders (notably sprue and iron-deficiency anemia) cause abnormal loss of copper.

Other trace elements are also widely available. Cobalt, an essential component of vitamin B_{12}, can be obtained from milk, muscle meats, and organ meats. Manganese, important to bone structure, reproduction, and the normal functioning of the central nervous system, is abundant in nuts, whole grains, and some legumes. Availability of selenium, a little-understood substance that is tentatively being linked to protein-calorie malnutrition, is dependent upon soil content in the region in which meats and grains have been produced. Chromium, possibly vital to normal glucose metabolism, is found in all animal protein (except fish), as well as in whole grain products and brewer's yeast.

These and many other micro-nutrients contribute to the overall health of man, yet their exact functions remain unknown,partially because no serious deficiency diseases have occurred to spur scientists into in-depth investigation of the exact roles played by the lesser-known trace elements. Unfortunately, dietary trace-element imbalances may someday occur if the use of highly processed, highly refined foods continues to increase. Though these foods may be fortified with major vitamins and minerals, they seldom contain trace elements in significant amounts.

Ironically, many consumers feel most confident when buying such products, since goverment-labeling mandates have forced manufacturers to let the public know the percentage of the recommended daily allowance of eight important vitamins and minerals that are available in a serving portion of such foods as puddings mixes and breakfast tarts. A woman is usually favorably impressed by the fact that a certain cereal features high percentages of the eight nutrients that must be listed on every label. She may not realize that the RDA referred to by these labels usually represents the *highest* RDA on the National Research Council's chart, approximately that for an adolescent boy. Since a woman's RDA of vitamins, minerals, and protein is often considerably less than that of an adolescent boy, she may well be taking an overdose of certain vitamins. Furthermore, a natural, whole-grain product, though unfortified with "Big 8" vitamins and minerals, may well be more vital to her overall health, because it contains several micronutrients that have been refined out of most heavily fortified cereals.

The woman who starts her day with a highly refined, vitamin-mineral-rich cereal, has a powdered high-vitamin, low-calorie packet stirred into eight ounces of milk for lunch, and heats up a preprocessed or frozen dinner may have consumed products with abundant supplies of the much-advertised nutrients appearing on package labels yet virtually devoid of important trace elements available in less highly refined yet equally nutritious foods. On the other hand, our environment is constantly bombarded with heavy metals and other such elements, many of which are finding their way into the food supply in ever-increasing amounts. Dietary decreases of some naturally occurring elements and increases of some elements not formerly appearing in the human diet in significant amounts are becoming increasingly common. The effect that such alterations of the natural distribution of trace elements will have on trace-element balance is yet to be seen.

For the pregnant woman who follows recommended daily dietary allowances for trace elements and eats enough meats, fish, and/or fresh vegetables to ensure adequate intakes of other micronutrients trace-element deficiency is highly unlikely.

MEETING THE NUTRITIONAL NEEDS OF PREGNANCY — UNDERSTANDING AND USING THE EXCHANGE PLAN

> The exchange system . . . is based upon a simple grouping of common foods according to generally equivalent nutritional values. This system may be used for any situation requiring calorie and food value control.
>
> Sue Rodwell Williams
> *(Nutrition and Diet Therapy,*
> C. V. Mosby Company, St. Louis, 1969)

Though RDA charts and paragraphs explaining the importance of various nutrients may convince a pregnant woman that she should be eating well-balanced meals, planning those meals may sometimes seem an impossible task and too technical. Most women don't fully understand an international unit or a mg, let alone know how to measure food in terms of such units. Preparing three meals that will contain just 1.3 mg of thiamin, 1.5 mg of riboflavin, .800 mg of folic acid, 15 IU of vitamin E, plus equally exacting measurements of other vital nutrients would tax the skills of a trained chemist. It would also take all the joy out of cooking and eating.

Fortunately, there's no need to be worried about *exact* measurements of vital nutrients. Eating meals that contain vitamin-A-rich vegetables and dairy products will mean eating around 5,000 IU of Vitamin A. RDA charts were derived at least in part from studies of the eating habits of the average healthy American. Furthermore, except for energy (calorie) recommendations all recommendations are set higher than the minimum necessary to maintain good health and avoid deficiency symptoms.

Except for those persons who continue to use fad diets, those who habitually eat highly refined, high-calorie, low-nutrition junk foods, or those with malabsorption or other serious medical disorders, pregnant women should be able to get all necessary protein, vitamins, and minerals in meals that the entire family can enjoy, meals that can be easily prepared once certain basic steps have been mastered. Assessment of calorie needs, the first step toward adequate nutrition, is one that should be taken early in pregnancy.

As mentioned earlier, energy needs vary from person to person, depending on such factors as activity, metabolism differences, and state of health. Nonetheless, the stated energy requirements of the National Research Council's "average pregnant woman" is a good starting point for most pregnant women, provided that energy intakes at this level result in an acceptable prenatal-weight-gain curve leading to a gain of approximately 24 pounds. A pregnant woman should meet the RDA calorie level shown in Chapter 4 (300 calories above the RDA for her age, weight, and height) and make adjustments up or down as she and her doctor view her weight-gain pattern.

Since energy requirements vary with age, a 33-year-old woman may gain too rapidly on a 2,300 calorie diet. Since such requirements are also affected by activity, a 20-year-old swimming instructor might find a 2,400 calorie diet provides insufficient gains. Assessing current caloric intakes, provided that intake has not led to an underweight state or to obesity, usually gives an idea of a woman's caloric maintenance level. Adding 300 calories to that intake to meet the energy demands of pregnancy will probably yield a workable calorie figure. Daily meal plans can easily be adjusted to fit the appropriate figure, using The Daily Meal Pattern Chart in this chapter.

Remember—*all* calories count, those taken in snacks or consumed as cocktails as well as those eaten during meals. At mealtime 2,300 calories, supplemented by a 250-calorie ice-cream sundae, means 2,550 calories. This probably means overnutrition with resultant obesity if a woman's maintenance + pregnancy calorie level should be 2,300. Plan snacks as well as meals, increasing the likelihood that such snacks will be nutritious and decreasing the possibility that thoughtlessly nibbled calories will push weight beyond desired limits.

Consuming 2,300 calories per day certainly does not guarantee adequate nutrition for a mother-to-be or for the child she carries. Overemphasis on empty calories such as highly refined sugars, pastas, and chips can mean adequate energy levels but inadequate levels of protein, vitamins, and minerals. To the doctor such a woman may appear fairly well-nourished, since the prenatal weight curve is steady and total weight gain equals 24 pounds or more. Unfortunately, the doctor cannot know which foods supplied the calories leading to these gains. Unless he discovers nutritional deficiencies severe enough to cause some outward evidence in the expectant mother, he is not likely to suggest dietary changes. Nonetheless, the mother's health and that of her child may be endangered, even while prenatal weight gains form an ideal curve.

To make sure that her calories have sufficient quality as well as quantity, a pregnant woman needs help in meal planning. With RDA charts, a calorie book, and information on vitamin, mineral, and protein content of foods she can laboriously determine her daily needs and translate those needs into meal plans, but with this method her work has just begun. She must now measure (and often weigh) each portion of food before consuming it or else be liable to significant calorie deviations. Even with the use of her handy pocket calculator, such operations are beyond the average person.

The Exchange System
Fortunately, there is an easier way to plan meals. Some years back the pressing need for an easy-to-use meal planning guide for diabetics led to the development of an "exchange list" in which foods are grouped according to generally equivalent nutritional values. In this plan foods are divided into six basic lists, with all foods within a given list having approximately the same calorie, protein, and fat values and containing similar minerals and vitamins. Foods within any one group may be substituted for other foods in that same group.

The latest Exchange List for Meal Planning of the American Diabetes Association, Inc., and the American Dietetic Association (in cooperation with the National Institute of Arthritis, Metabolism, and Digestive Disease, the National Heart and Lung Institute, and the National Institutes of Health, Public Health Service, United States Department of Health, Education and Welfare) reflects current theories on modification of fat intake as well as carbohydrate intake. This latest list even shows the difference in saturated and polyunsaturated fats and lists high-, medium-, and low-fat meats separately, a concession to the ever-growing concern about rising cholesterol levels and their link to heart and circulation disorders. The list also contains information on vitamin and mineral content of the foods listed, an invaluable aid for the pregnant woman conscious of the need for balanced intakes of these elements.

The Exchange Groups
Though the following exchange lists are loosely based on Exchange Lists for Meal Planning, they are *not* intended for use by diabetics. A pregnant woman's diet includes many items that a diabetic must avoid. The modified exchange lists are intended to give a realistic picture of the foods available to nondiabetic persons. Special emphasis has been placed on milk products and on high-vitamin fruits and vegetables. The six primary exchange lists contain head notes as to the calorie, carbohydrate, fat, and protein content of each group. These lists have been modified to make it easier to choose foods high in important vitamins and minerals and to include desserts and other items not usually seen on exchange lists but often used by healthy American women. Note: The *amounts* of each food item must be considered when you use the Daily Meal Planning Chart in this chapter. Each exchange list indicates the serving size equal to one exchange.

MILK EXCHANGE

Description	Service Size	Carbo-hydrate (g)	Protein (g)	Fat (g)	Calorie (kcal)
A. Nonfat	8 oz.	12	8	trace	80
B. Low-fat (2%)	8 oz.	12	8	2.5−5	102−125
C. Whole	8 oz.	12	8	10	170

Milk products, man's leading source of calcium, also provide protein, phosphorus, magnesium, zinc, and some B-complex vitamins (including folic acid and B_{12}). If fortified, they are high in vitamins A and D. Nonfat and 2%-low-fat milk products provide the above nutrients at a lower calorie cost than do whole-milk products. The Daily Meal Pattern Chart in this chapter takes into account the varied fat contents of the three types of milk products. In using that chart one must specify whether nonfat, low-fat, or whole-milk products are being used.

Milk groups	Amount equal to one exchange
A. Nonfat Fortified	
Skim or nonfat	1 cup
Powdered (before liquid)	1/3 cup
Canned-evaporated skim	½ cup
Skim-milk buttermilk	1 cup
Skim-milk yogurt (plain)	1 cup
B. Low-Fat Fortified	
1%	1 cup
2%	1 cup
2% yogurt (plain)	1 cup
2% chocolate milk (commercial)	1 cup
C. Whole	
Whole canned evaporated milk	½ cup
Buttermilk (whole)	1 cup
Yogurt (whole, plain)	1 cup
Malted milk	1 cup
Cocoa	1 cup
*Cheese	
Cottage cheese	½ cup (pressed down)
Cheddar cheese (natural)	1 oz. or ¼ cup grated, pressed down
Cheddar cheese (pasteurized, processed)	1 oz. or ¼ cup grated, pressed down
Parmesan (grated)	1 oz. or ¼ cup grated, pressed down
Swiss (natural)	1 oz. or ¼ cup grated, pressed down
Swiss (pasteurized, processed)	1 oz. or ¼ cup grated, pressed down
Ice milk	1 cup (enter one fat exchange)
Ice cream	1 cup (enter two fat exchanges)
Baked custard	1 cup (enter two fat exchanges)

*Other cheeses (camembert, blue roquefort, cream cheese, pasteurized processed cheese foods, and cheese spreads) contain calcium proportions much lower than milk. Since very large high-calorie servings would be needed to enable one to count these as milk, they should be considered as a protein source (meat exchange). The calcium content of creams (sour cream, whipping cream, half-and-half) is relatively low considering the number of calories that must be consumed to match the calcium content of 1 cup of 2% milk. They should be considered as fats for the purposes of an exchange diet.

VEGETABLE EXCHANGE

Description	Serving Size	Carbo-hydrate (g)	Protein (g)	Fat (g)	Calories (kcal)
A. Leafy green vegetables	as noted	5	2	—	25
B. Other vegetables	as noted	5	2	—	25
C. Vitamin-C-rich vegetables	as noted	5	2	—	25

A. Leafy green vegetables — high in vitamins A, E, B_6, B_9 (folic acid), riboflavin, iron, magnesium, and potassium

1 exchange = ½ cup, cooked   **1 exchange = any amount desired, raw**

Asparagus	Chicory
Bok choy	Endive
Broccoli	Escarole
Brussels sprouts	Lettuce: red leaf, iceberg, romaine
Cabbage	Parsley
Greens: beets, collards, dandelion, kale,	Sauerkraut
mustard, spinach, swiss chard, turnip	Watercress
Scallions (green onions)	Vegetable-juice cocktail

B. Other Vegetables — supply varied amounts of B-complex vitamins, vitamin E, magnesium, zinc, and phosphorus; carrots and summer squash are high sources of vitamin A.

1 exchange = ½ cup, cooked   **1 exchange = any amount desired, raw**

Artichoke	Cucumbers	Chinese cabbage
Bamboo shoots	Eggplant	Radishes
Bean sprouts	Mushrooms	
Alfalfa sprouts	Nori seaweed	
Mung	Okra	
Beets	Onion	
Burdock root	Rhubarb	
Carrots	String Beans: yellow, green	
Celery	Summer squash	
	Zucchini	

C. Vitamin-C-Rich Vegetables

1 exchange = ½ cup, cooked

Asparagus	Mustard
Bok choy	Swiss chard
Broccoli	Turnips
Brussels sprouts	Peppers: bell (green or red), chili
Cabbage	Rutabagas
Collard greens	Tomatoes
Kale	Tomato juice
Dandelion	Vegetable-juice cocktail

FRUIT EXCHANGE

Description	Serving Size	Carbo-hydrate (g)	Protein (g)	Fat (g)	Calories (kcal)
A. General fruits and juices	as noted	10	—	—	40
B. Vitamin-C-rich fruits and juices	as noted	10	—	—	40

Fruits may be used fresh, frozen, canned, dried, cooked, or raw as long as no sugar is added. Fruits provide significant amounts of vitamins (A, C, folic acid), minerals (iron and potassium), and fiber.
One exchange equals the serving size shown.

A. General fruits and juices

Apple, 1 small
Applesauce (unsweetened) ½ cup
Apricots, fresh*, 2 medium
Apricots, dried*, 4 halves
Banana, ½ small
Berries: blackberries, ½ cup;
   blueberries, ½ cup
Cherries, 10 large
Cranberries, 1 cup
Dates, 2 (1 cup = 12 fruit)
Figs (fresh or dried), 1
Grapes, 12
Watermelon, 1 cup
Nectarine*, 1 small
Peach*, 1 medium
Pear, 1 small
Persimmon (native)*, 1 medium
Pineapple, ½ cup
Plums, 2 medium
Prunes, 2 medium
Pumpkin*, 3½ oz. (raw)
Pumpkin, 2/5 cup (canned)
Raisins, 2 tablespoons (1 cup = 8 fruit)
Apple cider, 1/3 cup
Apple juice, 1/3 cup
Grape juice, ¼ cup
Pineapple juice, 1/3 cup
Prune juice, ¼ cup

B. Vitamin-C-rich fruits and juices

Raspberries, ½ cup
Strawberries, ¾ cup
Grapefruit, ½
Guava, ¼ medium
Mango*, ½ small
Cantaloupe*, ¼ small
Honeydew, 1/8 medium
Orange, 1 small
Papaya, ¾ cup
Tangerine, 1 medium
Grapefruit juice, ½ cup
Orange juice, ½ cup

High Vitamin-A content

Note: Apricots, bananas, berries, grapefruit, grapefruit juice, mangoes, cantaloupes, honeydews, nectarines, oranges, orange juice, and peaches are all rich in potassium. Oranges, orange juice, and cantaloupe provide folic acid.

BREADS AND STARCHY VEGETABLES

Description	Serving Size	Carbo-hydrate (g)	Protein (g)	Fat (g)	Calories (kcal)
A. Breads, cereals, crackers	as noted	15	2	—	70
B. Vegetables	as noted	15	2	—	70

Relatively high in carbohydrates, most items on this list are an excellent source of energy. *Moderate* reduction of high-carbohydrate foods enables one to lower total calorie load without risking loss of nutritional balance. Whenever possible, choose to retain items high in vitamins, minerals, and/or protein. One exchange is equal to the portion size shown.

Food	Serving size (equal to one exchange)
A. 1. Bread	
Bagel	½ cup
Dried bread crumbs	3 tablespoons
English muffin	½ small
French	1 slice
Frankfurter roll	½
Hamburger roll	½
Italian	1 slice
Plain roll	1
Pumpernickel	1 slice
Raisin	1 slice
Rye	1 slice
Tortilla	1, 6"
White	1 slice
Whole wheat	1 slice
2. Cereal	
Barley (cooked)	½ cup
Bran flakes	½ cup
Cereal, ready to eat, unsweetened	¾ cup
Cereal, puffed, unsweetened	1
Cornmeal (dry)	2 tablespoons
Farina (cooked)	½ cup
Flour*	2½ tablespoons
Grits (cooked)	½ cup
Pasta (cooked): macaroni, noodles, spaghetti	½ cup
Popcorn (popped, no fat added)	3 cups
Rice (cooked)	½ cup
Wheat germ	¼ cup

Flour: For recipe conversion, the following flour exchanges are useful. Use the same figures for plain, whole-wheat, rye or other flour:

    2 tablespoons = 1 bread exchange
    8 tablespoons = ½ cup = 4 bread exchanges
    16 tablespoons = 1 cup = 8 bread exchanges

Food	Serving size (equal to one exchange)
3. Crackers	
Arrowroot	3
Graham, 2½" square	2
Matzoh, 4" x 6"	½
Oyster	20
Pretzels, 3½" x 1/8"	25
Rye wafers, 2" x 3½"	3
Saltines	6
Soda, 2½" square	4
B. Vegetables (cooked)	
Baked beans (canned)	¼ cup
Corn	1/3 cup
Corn on cob	1 small
Dried beans	½ cup
Dried lentils	½ cup
Dried peas	½ cup
Lima beans	½ cup
Parsnips	2/3 cup
Peas, green (canned or frozen)	½ cup
Potato, sweet	¼ cup
Potato, white	1 small
Potato, mashed	½ cup
Pumpkin	¾ cup
Soybeans	½ cup
Winter squash (acorn or butternut)	½ cup
Yam	¼ cup

MEAT EXCHANGE

Description	Service Size	Carbo-hydrate (g)	Protein (g)	Fat (g)	Calorie (kcal)
A. Lean	as noted	—	7	3	55
B. Medium-fat	as noted	—	7	5.5	77
C. High-fat	as noted	—	7	8	100

All three meat categories contain foods that are good sources of protein. Many of the animal-origin foods on the list also provide significant amounts of iron, zinc, and several B-complex vitamins. Group A, lean meats, is recommended for those wishing to avoid high cholesterol levels. Peanut butter, a vegetable food from list B, is high in fat yet contains no cholesterol. The Daily Meal Pattern Chart takes into account the varied fat content of foods on the three meat-exchange lists. In using that chart one must specify whether lean, medium-fat, or high-fat meats are being used.

	Amount equal to one exchange

A. Lean Meat

Beef: baby beef (very lean), chipped beef, chuck, flank steak, tenderloin, plate ribs, plate skirt steak, round (bottom or top), rump (all cuts), spare ribs, tripe	1 ounce
Lamb: leg, rib, sirloin, loin (roast and chops), shank, shoulder	1 ounce
Pork: leg (whole rump, center shank), ham (smoked center slice)	1 ounce
Veal: leg, loin, rib, shank, shoulder, cutlets	1 ounce
Poultry: chicken, turkey, Cornish hen, guinea hen, pheasant (all without skin)	1 ounce
Fish: fresh, frozen, or canned salmon, tuna, mackerel	1 ounce
crab, lobster	¼ cup
clams, oysters, scallops, shrimp	1 ounce or 5 pcs.
sardines (drained)	3
Cheese with less than 5% butterfat*	1 ounce
Cottage cheese, dry and 2% butterfat*	¼ cup
Dried beans and peas (omit one bread exchange)	½ cup

B. Medium-fat meat

Beef: ground (15% fat), corned beef (canned), ribeye, round (ground commercial)	1 ounce
Pork: loin (all cuts tenderloin), shoulder arm (picnic), shoulder blade, Boston butt, Canadian bacon, boiled ham	1 ounce
Variety meats: liver, heart, kidney, sweetbreads (high in cholesterol)	1 ounce
Cheese: cottage (creamed),	¼ cup
mozzarella, ricotta, farmer's cheese, neufchatel,	1 ounce
parmesan*	3 tablespoons
Egg (high in cholesterol)	1
Peanut butter (omit two extra fat exchanges)	2 tablespoons

C. High-fat Meat

Beef: brisket, corned beef (brisket), ground beef (about 20% fat), hamburger (commercial), chuck (ground commercial), roast (rib), steaks (club and rib)	1 ounce
Lamb: breast	1 ounce
Pork: spare ribs, loin (back ribs), pork (ground), country-style ham, deviled ham**	1 ounce
Veal: breast	1 ounce
Poultry: capon, duck (domestic), goose	1 ounce
Cheese: cheddar types*	1 ounce
Cold cuts: ½" x 1/8" slice	4
Frankfurter	1 small

*Some cheeses are high in calcium and can count toward daily milk quotas (see milk exchange list); they do *not* supply iron
**Bacon is listed on the fat-exchange list

FAT EXCHANGES

Description	Serving Size	Carbo-hydrate (g)	Protein (g)	Fat (g)	Calories (kcal)
A. Polyunsaturated	as noted	—	—	5	45
B. Monounsaturated	as noted	—	—	5	45
C. Saturated	as noted	—	—	5	45

Both animal and vegetable fats are concentrated calorie sources and should be used in moderation. Those persons wishing to avoid high cholesterol intakes should avoid saturated fats. Polyunsaturated fats have been associated with decreases in blood cholesterol.

	Amount equal to one exchange
A. Polyunsaturated Fats	
*Margarine: soft, tub, or stick (made with corn,	1 teaspoon
cottonseed, safflower, soy, or sunflower oil)	
Oil: corn, cottonseed, safflower, soy, sunflower	1 teaspoon
Walnuts (½ cup = 16 fat)	6 small
Dressing: French, Italian (if made with corn, cottonseed,	1 tablespoon
safflower, soy, or sunflower oil)	
Mayonnaise-type salad dressing (if made with	2 teaspoons
corn, cottonseed, safflower, soy, or sunflower oil)	
Mayonnaise (if made with corn, cottonseed, safflower,	1 teaspoon
soy, or sunflower oil)	
B. Monounsaturated Fats	
Avocado (4" in diameter)	1/8
Oil: olive, peanut	1 teaspoon
Olives	5 small
Almonds (½ cup = 15 fat)	10 whole
Pecans (½ cup = 17 fat)	2 large
Peanuts (½ cup = 15 fat); Spanish	20 whole
Virginia	19 whole
Sesame seeds (½ cup = 14 fat)	1 tablespoon
Other nuts	6 small

*For recipe conversion the following margarine or butter exchanges are useful:

1/8 stick = 1 tablespoon = 3 fat exchanges
¼ stick = 1/8 cup = 3 tablespoons = 6 fat exchanges
½ stick = ¼ cup = 4 tablespoons = 12 fat exchanges
2/3 stick = 1/3 cup = 5½ tablespoons = 16½ fat exchanges
¼ pound = 1 stick = ½ cup = 8 tablespoons = 24 fat exchanges
½ pound = 2 sticks = 1 cup = 16 tablespoons = 48 fat exchanges

C. Saturated Fats**

Margarine, regular stick (made from animal fat)	1 teaspoon
Butter	1 teaspoon
Bacon fat .	1 teaspoon
Bacon, crisp-fried	1 strip
Coconut	2-3 tablespoons
Cream, light	2 tablespoons
Cream, sour	2 tablepoons
Cream, heavy	1 tablespoon
Cream cheese	1 tablespoon
Nondairy creamers**	5 tablespoons
Salt pork	¾" cube
Lard	1 teaspoon

**Anything made with coconut oil is high in saturated fats.

FREE EXCHANGES

In addition to the items included on the six exchange lists a number of other items may be included in a daily meal plan without restriction. These free exchanges include certain foods and almost all spices.

Beverages and foods

Coffee
Tea
Club soda
Clear broth
Clam juice
Bouillion (nonfat)
Low-cal soft drinks
Lemon
Unsweetened gelatin
Unsweetened cranberries
Unsweetened pickles

Spices and flavorings

Salt
Pepper
Herbs
Dry mustard
Chili powder
Cacao (dry)
Red or white horseradish
Lemon and lime juice
Soy sauce
Worchestershire sauce
Dehydrated onion flakes
Pure or natural extracts (lemon, maple, vanilla)
Saccharin and other noncaloric sweeteners (unless doctor advises against them)

Prepared Foods

Several commonly used prepared foods are shown below. The indicated serving size of these foods is equal to the number and type of exchanges shown. Enter each exchange in its proper column on the meal pattern chart.

Food	Serving Size	Exchange
A. Breads		
Banana	1 slice (3" x 3" x ½")	1½ bread, 1 fat
Biscuit	1 (2" diameter)	1 bread, 1 fat
Corn	1 piece (2" x 2" x 1')	1 bread, 1 fat
Corn muffin	1 (2" diameter)	1 bread, 1 fat
Crackers (round butter type)	5	1 bread, 1 fat
Croutons (no fat added)	1 cup	1 bread
Doughnuts (cake type, plain)	1	1 bread, 1 fat
Muffin:		
plain, blueberry	1 (average size)	1 bread, 1 fat
Pancakes	1 (5" x ½")	1 bread, 1 fat
Raisin	1 slice	1 bread
Taco shell:		
corn, ready-to-eat	1 (5½" diameter)	1 bread, 1 fat
corn, not fried	1 (6" diameter)	1 bread
flour, not fried	1 (7" diameter)	1 bread, 1 fat
Waffles	1 (5" x ½")	1 bread, 1 fat
B. Desserts		
Cake:		
angel, no icing	1/20 (1½" slice	1 bread
cupcake, no icing	1	1½ bread, 1 fat
mix, no icing	1/12 cake	1¼ bread, ½ fat
pound, no icing	1 (3" x 3" x ½")	1 bread, 1 fat
sponge, no icing	1/20 (1½")	1 bread
Cookies (high in fruit, nuts, and whole grains and low in sugar)		
Fig newton	2 (average)	1½ bread
Ginger snaps	5 (small)	1 bread
Oatmeal raisin	2 (small)	1½ bread
Peanut butter	2 (small)	1 bread, 1 fat
Chocolate chip	2 (small)	1½ bread
Date cookies	2 (small)	1½ bread
Custard	See milk-exchange list	
Ice cream	See milk-exchange list	
Piecrust (shell only)		
graham-cracker	⅛ of 9" pie	½ bread, 1½ fat
pastry	⅛ of 9" pie	½ bread, 1 fat
Pudding (regular, cooked, and instant)		
whole-milk	½ cup	1½ bread, ½ whole milk
skim-milk	½ cup	1½ bread, ½ skim milk
Sherbet	¼ cup	1 bread
Whipped topping (2% milk)	5 tablespoons	1 fat, 1/5 2% milk
C. Soups, Sauces, Snacks		
Cheese sauce	¼ cup	½ bread, ½ whole milk, 1½ fat
Gravy (made with flour)	2 tablespoons	1 fat
Hollandaise sauce	¼ cup	½ meat, 3 fat
Tartar sauce	1 tablespoon	2 fat
White sauce	2 tablespoons	1 fat
Corn chips	15	1 bread, 2 fat

Potato chips	15	1 bread, 2 fat
French fries	8 (2" to 3½")	1 bread, 1 fat
Cheddar-cheese soup (diluted)	1 cup	¼ bread, ½ whole milk
Cheddar-cheese soup (undiluted)	1 can (10¾ ounce)	¾ bread, 1¼ whole milk, 2½ fat
Cream-of-celery soup (diluted)*	1 cup	½ bread, 1 fat
Cream-of-celery soup (undiluted)	1 can (10¾ ounce)	1 bread, 2½ fat
Cream-of-chicken soup (diluted)	1 cup	½ bread, 1 fat
Cream-of-chicken soup (undiluted)	1 can (10¾ ounce)	1 bread, 2½ fat
Cream-of-mushroom soup (diluted)	1 cup	½ bread, 2 fat
Cream-of-mushroom (undiluted)	1 can (10¾ ounce)	2 bread, 4 fat
Tomato soup (diluted)	1 cup	1 bread, ½ fat
Tomato soup (undiluted)	1 can (10¾ ounce)	2½ bread, 1¼ fat

diluted means ½ soup, ½ water

Simple Carbohydrates

The following items provide energy but have little nutritional value. Honey or brown sugar may be substituted for white granulated sugar to achieve variety of flavor, but there is no nutritional advantage to such substitution. Molasses contains a significant amount of iron. The simple carbohydrate exchanges are expressed as breads, yet they should *not* be exchanged for one of the minimum required breads from the nucleus list of daily exchanges. They may count as additional breads beyond the minimum number of bread exchanges.

Carbohydrate	Exchange
Jam or jelly	1 tablespoon = ¾ bread exchange
Molasses	1 tablespoon = ½ bread exchange
	1 cup = 8 bread exchanges
Table syrups	1 tablespoon = 1 bread exchange
	1 cup = 8 bread exchanges
Sugar (white, granulated, or brown)	1 tablespoon = 2/3 bread exchange
	1 cup = 11 bread exchange
Sugar (powdered)	1 cup = 6½ bread exchanges
Honey	1 tablespoon = 2/3 bread exchange
	1 cup = 10 bread exchanges

Beverages (non-nutritional)

The following beverages contribute significant amounts of calories and little or no protein, vitamins, and minerals. Though expressed as bread and fat exchanges, they must not be used as substitutes for the minimum bread exchanges recommended on each day's meal-pattern chart.

Beverage	Serving Size	Exchange
A. Alcoholic		
Beer (4.5% alcohol)	12 fluid ounces	1 bread, 2 fats
Brandy or cognac	1 fluid ounce	1½ fat
Liquor (gin, rum, scotch, vodka, whiskey)	1½ fluid ounces	3 fat
Port wine	3½ fluid ounces	1 bread, 2 fat
Sherry, dry	2 fluid ounces	¼ bread, 1½ fat
Wine, dry table (12%)	3½ fluid ounces	¼ bread, 1½ fat
B. Nonalcoholic		
Cola (any regular)	3 fluid ounces	¾ bread
Ginger ale	4 fluid ounces	¾ bread

The Meal-Pattern Chart

No one of the above exchange groups can provide all the nutrients essential to a well-balanced diet. Planning a 2,400-calorie diet involves combining items from each list into attractive, sensible meals plus snacks for a total yield of 2,400 calories. To make such combinations simpler, a Daily Meal Pattern Chart for a 2,400-calorie diet appears on the next page. By adding or subtracting items a mother-to-be can lower or raise the calorie level to meet her own needs. Since this pattern may not appeal to some women while others may need to adapt this diet to fit special medical needs, a blank chart has been included in the Appendix. By following the steps supplied there a woman can design her own meal patterns to fit her personal calorie needs. If medical problems are involved, she should seek the help of a nutritional counselor and/or her physician in planning her meal pattern.

Adjusting Calorie Levels

Since the Daily Meal Pattern Chart on the following pages is designed for a 2,400 calorie diet, some woman will need to raise or lower the calorie load to fit their own needs. In adding or subtracting items from the meal pattern chart one must be sure to leave in the daily minimums of each exchange. If these minimums are not met, the diet will not meet RDA standards for protein, vitamins, and minerals. In general, to adjust the Daily Meal Pattern Chart, a pregnant woman should add high-protein foods, milk products, fruits, or vegetables and deduct fats, simple carbohydrates, and high-calorie bread items.

By using the Daily Meal Pattern Chart and the exchange lists to which it refers a pregnant woman can plan delicious, well-balanced menus to meet her own needs, those of her unborn child, and those of her husband and other family members. Her husband's calorie needs probably equal or exceed her own, and the foods prepared according to the meal pattern chart will enable him to meet those needs in the optimum manner. Though the caloric needs of young children may be lower than those of a pregnant woman, their protein, vitamin, and mineral needs are similar enough that this basic meal pattern chart need hardly be altered to fit their needs and appetites. Turning the meal planning chart into menus is not difficult if one remembers that the chart is intended to be flexible. A woman can achieve great variety by trying many different vegetables, fruits, meats, and breads. The exchange lists allow her to determine which items may be exchanged or substituted without the risk of falling below RDA standards.

Many women prefer to obtain their calcium by eating milk products rather than by drinking milk. Since many dairy products are high in calcium, this alternative is perfectly acceptable, *provided that* the additional fat and/or carbohydrate content of these foods is considered in planning the total day's exchanges. For example, one cup of ice cream can count as one eight-ounce serving of whole milk but must also count as *one extra fat exchange.*

Bread exchanges gained through desserts are most beneficial if they contain whole grains, fruits, and minimum amounts of sugar. Choosing a fig newton over a sugar cookie makes good nutrition sense, because the former offers iron as well as carbohydrates. In general, choose cookies, cakes, and custards that offer more than just calories.

Converting Recipes To Exchange Values

Designing menus that follow the meal-pattern chart is simple as long as one uses foods whose exchange values appear on the exchange lists. If vegetables, fruits, milk products, meats, and most breads are served in simple form, their values are easy to determine. If food items from separate lists are combined in casseroles, desserts, or other dishes, exchange values of individual portions must be calculated by analyzing the recipe used. Exchange values for some commonly used prepared foods appear earlier in this chapter. Several publications featuring more extensive lists of exchange values for prepared foods are listed in the Bibliography.

More and more cookbooks include exchange values for each recipe. However, these books are often limited to recipes that are especially well suited to persons with health problems. Since a pregnant woman is not likely to want to limit herself to recipes of this sort, she should learn to calculate exchange values for her favorite recipes. If she notes these values on an index card or in the cookbook in which the recipe appears, she will soon build a collection of

DAILY MEAL PATTERN CHART FOR 2400 CALORIE PRENATAL DIET

	MILK A 80	MILK B 125	MILK C 170	Milk Kcal Per Meal Or Snack	VEG A 25	VEG B 25	VEG C 25	Vegetable Kcal Per Meal Or Snack	FRUIT A 40	FRUIT B 40	Fruit Kcal Per Meal Or Snack	BREAD A 70	BREAD B 70	Bread Kcal Per Snack	MEAT A 55	MEAT B 77	MEAT C 100	Meat Kcal Per Meal Or Snack	FAT 45	Fat Kcal Per Meal Or Snack	Total Kcal Per Meal Or Snack
Breakfast		1½		188					1		40	2		140		1	1	177	2	90	635
Mid-morning Snack													1	70		1		77			147
Lunch		1		125	1	1		50	1		40	2		140		2		154	2	90	599
Afternoon Snack																					
Dinner		1½		188	1		1	50	2		80	3	1	280		4		308	2	90	996
Evening Snack									1		40										40
Actual Daily Totals Per Exchange		4		501	2	1	1	100	3	2	200	8	1	630		8	1	716	6	270	2417
Recommended Minimum Daily Totals	4			varies 320-680	2			75	1		40	3	1	280	8-9			varies 495-900	as needed to meet calorie requirements		Maximum 2400 Calories

recipes keyed to the exchange system. The Conversion Chart which follows this section gives four basic steps for converting recipes to exchange values plus a sample recipe conversion.

A table of portion equivalents for meats is included in case one cannot weigh meat portions. Exchange values for soups and sauces commonly used in recipes have already been given. When in doubt, make an intelligent guess based on available data. Since a relatively small proportion of a day's exchanges will be based on guesswork, slight errors should not be too serious. Most cans list ounces and calories, and one can usually assign exchange values based on these two values. While one may not get the exchanges exactly right, they should at least yield the right number of calories.

In looking up recipe ingredients on the exchange list use logic and/or the process of elimination to determine which list to consult. For example, egg, a protein food, appears on the meat-exchange list: it is not a milk, vegetable, fruit, fat, or bread. Do not give up if the food does not appear on the first list consulted. Potato is not on the vegetable list, but it is on the starchy-vegetable section of the bread-exchange list. Sour cream does not appear as a milk product, but it does appear on the fat-exchange list.

With practice one can correctly guess which list to consult. With more practice exchange values for commonly used items can be recalled from memory. The system is not complicated, but it does require familiarity. Since the exchange method can become a lifetime way of meeting a family's nutritional needs, learning to use the method is well worth the effort.

Portion Equivalents and Measures
3 ounces of cooked meat (3 meat exchanges) are equal to:
    4 ounces lean, raw meat or fish without skin or bone
    ¾ cup cooked, flaked, or diced meat, poultry, or fish
    2 slices dark or light *cooked* turkey, 4½" x 2" x ¼" each
    ½ large chicken breast, cooked (without skin)
    1 chicken leg plus thigh, cooked (without skin)
    2 lean lamb chops (cooked) 3¾" x 2" x ½" each
    1 lean pork chop (cooked) 3¾" x 2" x ⅜"
2 ounces of cooked meat (2 meat exchanges) are equal to:
    1 serving veal 2½" x 3" x ½" (roasted or baked)
    1 hamburger patty 2½" in diameter x ½" thick (raw)
    5 1" cubes of stew meat (raw)

Planning Menus and Snacks
Once a woman has learned to convert recipes to exchange values, she is ready to plan daily menus and snacks. Keeping in mind the basic patterns described in the meal pattern chart, she merely fills in dishes that fit those patterns fairly well. For example, the breakfast pattern and a breakfast menu appear below.

CONVERSION CHART OF RECIPES TO EXCHANGE VALUES

	Step 1	Step 2	Step 3	Step 4
Instructions:	List all ingredients for the chosen recipe	To the right of this list note the exchange value of each ingredient	Determine the number of portions that the recipe makes and divide each exchange by that number	Consolidate the items (as shown below) to obtain exchange values for one portion of the recipe
Sample recipe conversion:	3 medium chicken breasts, halved and skinned	*24 meat exchanges	÷ 6 = 4 lean-meat exchanges	3 fat exchanges
	6 strips bacon	6 fat exchanges	÷ 6 = 1 fat exchange	
	1 jar dried beef (2½ ounce)	2½ lean-meat exchanges	÷ 6 = ½ lean-meat exchange	negligible bread exchange
	½ pint sour cream (8 ounces)	8 fat exchanges	÷ 6 = 1-1/3 fat exchange	
	1 can mushroom soup	**2 bread, 4 fat exchanges	÷ 6 = 1/3 bread, 2/3 fat exchange	4½ lean-meat exchanges

*Since the exchange value of meats and some vegetables is based on *cooked* amounts, you will need to adjust amounts by assuming that 1 pound of raw meat yields ¾ pound of cooked meat. For vegetables make adjustments only if there is a marked size increase or decrease after cooking. Since *exact* measurements are not crucial, using the chart of portion equivalents will make determining exchange values simpler.

**Items such as canned soups can be difficult to assess, unless one consults special exchange-list supplements found in relevant publications (see Bibliography).

BREAKFAST

Breakfast Pattern	Exchange Allowed	Exchange Used	Exchanges over or under	Breakfast Menu
Milk exchange B	1½	1	−½	8-ounce glass milk (2%)
Fruit exchange B	1	1	0	4-ounce orange juice
Bread exchange	2	2½	+½	1 English muffin (½ with 2 teaspoons jam, ½ plain)
Medium-fat meat exchange B	1	1	0	1 poached egg* (served on English muffin half)
High-fat meat exchange C	1	1**	0	1-ounce country-style ham
Fat exchange	2	1	−1	Butter for English muffin

*Women on low-cholesterol diets might substitute a scrambled low-cholesterol egg product.
**Since 1 ounce high-fat ham equals 100 calories and 2 ounces low-fat, center-slice smoked ham equals only 110 calories, the 2 ounces of low-fat meat might be substituted to give more protein and less fat with no significant calorie difference.

A quick inventory of the breakfast exchanges used shows carryover exchanges of milk (½ exchange) and fat (1 exchange) and an overcharge of bread (½ exchange). Slight alterations in the allowances for the day's other meals and/or snacks will take care of these variations form the breakfast pattern. In reality the bread and fat variation almost offset one another (in terms of calories) and need not be a cause for concern. Since the missing ½ milk exchange is needed to meet the recommended minimum milk quota, it must be accounted for at some point during the day.

Since planning the three meals, and adding snacks as they are needed to help meet quotas, seems a logical method of filling in the day's menu sheet, lunch is next to be considered. By writing in the lunch pattern, then consulting the exchange list a menu can be formed as shown below.

The missing Vitamin-C vegetable was eaten at lunch (the tomato in the chef's salad). Dinner gained ½ vegetable B, a negligible amount (12½ calories) of a vegetable not included in the dinner pattern of the meal-pattern chart. Other items are close enough to the pattern with two exceptions. The above dinner menu is quite high in fats, pushing the evening meal's fat consumption 2½ exchanges (about 113 calories) over the recommended level. This poses no great problem, provided that those calories are eliminated from some other part of the day's food intake. Skipping the morning bread and meat snack more than makes up for the fat calories accumulated at dinner, and with adequate protein (meat) and bread portions already planned for, skipping this meat/bread snack is perfectly acceptable. The second problem posed by the gourmet evening meal

LUNCH

Lunch Pattern	Exchange Allowed	Exchange Used	Exchanges over or under	Lunch Menu
Milk Exchange B	1	1½	+½	1 cup ice milk
Vegetable exchange A	1	1	0	Large chef's salad* with thousand-island dressing (4 teaspoons)
Vegetable exchange B	1	1	1	
Fruit exchange A	1	0	−1	
Breads	2	1	−1	3 rye wafers
Medium-fat meat B	2	1	−1	Iced tea (free exchange)
Fat	2	2½	+½	

*The recipe must be converted to exchange values, and those values can be entered under "exchange used." This salad, made to serve one person, contained:

    1 boiled egg = 1 medium-fat exchange
    ½ ounce cheddar cheese (grated) = ½ milk plus ½ fat exchange
    generous amounts of endive and iceberg lettuce = 1 vegetable-A exchange
    ½ cup chopped celery = 1 vegetable-B exchange
    1 small tomato = 1 vegetable-C exchange
    4 teaspoons of thousand-island dressing = 2 fat exchanges

In this case the cheese in the chef's salad provided the milk and fat exchanges missing from breakfast. The breakfast bread overcharge is offset by an undercharge at lunch, leaving ½ bread exchange to be eaten at some other time. An extra vegetable vlaue (tomato, a C vegetable) was used in the chef's salad and need not be used later.

After a salad lunch a gourmet dinner is a logical possibility. For easy calculation the main dish will be Party Chicken, the recipe whose exchange value was figured in the Conversion Chart earlier.

is its milk shortage. To make up for this shortage, one might have ½ cup cottage cheese and a small pear as a mid-morning snack and drink ½ cup 2% chocolate milk at bedtime or add the missing 4 ounces of milk to tomorrow's menu plan. The entire menu with snacks would appear as follows.

Although the above daily menu sheet deviates slightly from the meal-pattern chart in the arrangement of foods, it includes *all basic foods* in the amounts recommended and falls within the 2,400-calorie range (+100 cal).

Though the first planning of a daily menu that follows the meal-pattern chart may seem a bit difficult, each day's planning becomes easier. Soon a woman will be able to recall many exchange values from memory. She will also become increasingly more aware of which foods should go together to form a well-balanced diet. By the end of seven to nine months a pregnant woman should have mastered the art of planning well-balanced meals, an art that she can practice for many years to come.

DINNER

Dinner Pattern	Exchange Allowed	Exchange Used	Exchanges over or under	Dinner Menu
Milk B	1½	0	−1½	Party chicken (see Part III) for exchanges of fat and lean meat per serving
Vegetable A	1	1	0	½ cup wild rice (½ bread)
Vegetable C	1	0	−1	½ cup carrot-raisin salad (1 vegetable A, ½ fruit A)
Fruit A	2	½ + ¼	−¼	Green peas, onions, mushrooms (½ vegetable B, 1 bread)
Bread A	3	½ + ¹/₃ + 1	−¹/₃	Sour-cream cake (1 bread, 1½ fat)
Bread B	1	1	0	Cranapple topping (1/3 bread, ¼ fruit A)
Medium-fat meat B	4	4½	+½	
Fat	2	3 + 1½	+2½	

MENUS AND SNACKS FOR 2,400-CALORIE PRENATAL DIET

Breakfast:
: 8 ounces 2% milk
4 ounces orange juice
1 poached egg on ½ buttered English muffin
½ buttered English muffin with 2 teaspoon jam or jelly
1 ounce country-style ham or 2 ounces lean, center-slice smoked ham

Mid-morning snack:
: ½ cup cottage cheese
1 small pear

Lunch:
: Large chef's salad with 4 tablespoons thousand-island dressing (lettuce, endive, grated cheese, tomato, celery, egg)
3 rye wafers
1 glass iced tea
1 cup ice milk

Afternoon snack:
: —

Dinner:
: Party chicken (½ breast)*
Wild rice (½ cup)
Carrot-raisin salad (½ cup)*
Green peas/onions/mushrooms (½ cup)*
Iced tea
Sour-cream cake with cranapple topping*

Evening snack:
: ½ cup 2% chocolate milk

Recipe appears in Part III.

To make those first few days of meal planning a bit easier, a full week of daily menu plans appears in Part III. These 10 plans may be used as they are presented or altered according to the previously discussed directions for menu planning. When specific recipes are mentioned, they appear with an asterisk(*), an indication that the recipe, complete with exchange values, appears at the end of this book. Variations of the daily menus can be alternated with orignal daily menu plans until the homemaker gains more speed and expertise in menu planning. Once she has mastered this valuable skill, planning and preparing nutritious meals can become easier than throwing together haphazard last-minute specials.

The 7 sample daily menus are based on the 2,400-calorie Daily Meal Pattern Chart. Additional exchanges may be added by the woman who needs more calories, and the appropriate number of exchanges may be omitted by the woman who needs fewer calories. Remember to consult the recommended-minimum-daily-totals line to avoid omitting any nucleus foods. By using the menus that feature recipes included in this book a woman can become familiar with the exchange system without needing to learn how to convert recipes into exchanges. She may gradually add recipes of her own choosing, converting them to exchange values by using the steps in the Conversion Charts.

Once meal planning becomes a way of life for a pregnant woman, she's not likely to give it up; Thus the unborn child is doubly ensured against nutritional deficiencies. A good prenatal diet makes a good postpartum diet more likely, and a good postpartum diet probably means an excellent chance for the planning of nutritious meals to become a lifetime practice.

MEETING THE NUTRITIONAL NEEDS OF PREGNANCY: DIETARY TIPS FOR SPECIFIC COMPLAINTS

The so-called minor discomforts of pregnancy are the common complaints experienced by most expectant mothers, in the course of a normal pregnancy . . . They are not serious but their presence detracts from the mother's feeling of comfort and well-being. In many instances they can be avoided or entirely overcome by common sense in daily living.

Elise Fitzpatrick, RN, Nicholson J. Eastman, MD, and Sharan R. Reeder, RN, *Maternity Nursing, 11th edition,* J. B. Lippincott Company, Philadelphia, 1966)

What good are plans for a delicious breakfast if a pregnant woman's morning sickness means that breakfast is impossible? Fourtunately, morning sickness doesn't usually extend past the first three months of pregnancy, but those weeks of nausea are one of the most talked-about signs of pregnancy. For morning sickness and several other common discomforts of pregnancy there are food tips that may be of help.

Nausea and Vomiting

The most common disorder of pregnancy, nausea, or morning sickness, may actually occur at any time of the day. Appearing about the fifth or sixth week of pregnancy and ranging in severity from a slightly uneasy feeling to uncontrollable vomiting, this nausea is experienced by about 50% of pregnant women. While cases of severe vomiting may lead to liver damage, dehyration, acidosis, or other such complications, most reports of nausea describe mild discomfort, with only about one-third of the nausea victims experiencing vomiting.

The nausea usually occurs as a woman gets out of bed, lasts through early morning, and disappears by noon. Occasionally afternoon sickness or evening sickness is experienced instead. Except in severe cases the nausea has usually stopped by the 12th to 15th week, causing no permanent damage to the mother-to-be or to the fetus. Should unusually severe symptoms persist, a woman should ask her physician's advice. Just as in any case of severe, prolonged vomiting, there is danger of starvation and dehydration if treatment is not administered.

Some physicians have administered Vitamin B6 (pyridoxine) and reported good results, but others have found this treatment ineffective. Drugs are generally to be avoided because of possible damage to the fetus, though physicians do prescribe antinauseants or sedatives in severe cases. As with any use of drugs during pregnancy, a woman should not self-prescribe. The Thalidomide tragedy of the 1950s has made the risks of using drugs during pregnancy well known. A pregnant woman should ask her doctor to explain possible risks of any antinauseant drug that she is about to take.

In the case of morning sickness understanding that the nausea is fairly temporary and quite normal during pregnancy may help a woman to weather its unpleasant effects. Certain hormone changes may trigger a feeling of nausea in pregnant women similar to that experienced by some women while using oral contraceptives. Many doctors believe that the nausea is partly psychological, caused by the tensions brought about by the new situation of pregnancy. Nevertheless the sensation is real and unpleasant, and lessening its effects becomes a primary concern of the sufferer.

Coping with morning sickness means rescheduling one's early-morning meal. Since the nausea of pregnancy is more likely to occur on an empty stomach, with the first wave striking just as the woman sits up in bed or stands for the first time, many doctors recommend eating a slice of dry toast or a cracker or two before getting out of bed. For some a sip of hot tea or hot water with lemon juice may work well, but for most a *dry* start is essential. After half an hour has passed, get up very slowly, dress slowly, and avoid any sudden movements.

For women who are fine until they sit down at the breakfast table the crackers-in-bed routine can be skipped, but *dry* foods first are still advised. For example, a dry breakfast of a boiled egg and dry toast with jelly may be followed later in the morning by a liquid breakfast of citrus juice and milk with coffee or tea if desired. For the working woman the coffee break can become a second breakfast. If nausea persists throughout the day, all meals and snacks can follow this dry-first, liquid-second pattern, with meals being stretched out into five or six snacks rather than lumped into three big meals. Remember— fasting only makes nausea worse; eating small snacks at two- to three-hour intervals is wise, even if the thought of food isn't exciting!

Since maintaining an adequate energy supply is crucial, carbohydrates such as crackers or dry popcorn can be eaten. During severe bouts of morning sickness keeping down easily digested carbohydrates is more important than eating and then vomiting up hard-to-digest, high-protein foods. Worrying over lack of protein at a time when the body cannot readily digest it is useless.

Only in severe cases of persistent, prolonged vomiting (hyperemesis) does morning sickness cause serious problems—provided that a woman avoids the temptation to use over-the-counter antinausea drugs and makes every effort to see that an adequate energy supply is made available to her body.

The washed-out feeling of early pregnancy is often related to lack of energy. Following the necessary steps for control of nausea usually means increasing the energy supply and regaining strength, though extra rest periods may be needed to help a woman combat the low-energy fatigue. A quick-energy drink such as weak lemonade, ginger ale, or Coke, sipped after vomiting, sometimes helps.

Heartburn

While morning sickness is a complaint of early pregnancy, heartburn may occur at any time during the nine months of gestation. Often described as a burning sensation behind the lower part of the sternum, or breastbone, heartburn indicates irritation of the lining of the esophagus, which is caused by regurgitation of the stomach contents into the esophagus. In spite of its name heartburn has nothing to do with the heart.

Swallowing a tablespoon of cream or a pat of butter before meals may help to prevent an attack, since the fat counteracts the acid secretion in the stomach. This is a preventive means, not a treatment, since the cream has no effect after

COMBATING MORNING SICKNESS

Before rising	2 crackers or dry toast
½ an hour later	Slowly rise, dress, and prepare a "dry breakfast"
Breakfast-time	Eat a hard-boiled or soft-boiled egg and a slice of dry toast with jelly. NO LIQUIDS
Midmorning or coffee break	Have a "liquid breakfast" of milk, citrus juice, and coffee or tea if desired
Lunch and Dinner	As usual, unless nausea persists, in which case try a dry-liquid pattern similar to that of breakfast. Saving the beverage for a snack often works well

General Hints: Start with easy-to-digest carbohydrates, avoiding greasy fried foods, pastries, and rich desserts. Gradually move toward a "soft" diet, then a normal one.

heartburn occurs. Some physicians suggest avoiding fluids with meals to prevent diluting digestive juices. If this preventive measure is tried, one must be sure to take in adequate fluids between meals.

As in the case of morning sickness a woman should be careful to avoid over-the-counter medication. Even if a self-prescribed remedy proves harmless to the fetus, it may worsen the symptoms of heartburn, not lessen them. For instance, a sodium-bicarbonate (baking-soda) preparation is a "remedy" to be avoided, since some doctors feel that the sodium ion, taken in excess, may promote water retention. Furthermore, since sodium bicarbonates *increase* acid production before neutralizing stomach acids, they may cause considerable additional gastric distress. Once they have effectively neutralized stomach acids, they block absorption of certain minerals that require an acid environment in order to be used by the body. A pregnant woman should ask her doctor's advice if medication seems necessary. An aluminum-hydroxide gel or tablets containing magnesium trisilicate may prove helpful.

Flatulence

Flatulence often accompanies heartburn. If excessive gas is trapped in the stomach, belching may relieve symptoms. Pains caused by gas trapped in the intestinal tract may be relieved by the passing of flatus. Since neither belching nor breaking wind is an acceptable means of gas relief in company, prevention of gas buildup should be considered.

Swallowing excessive amounts of air may lead to increased flatulence. To avoid gulping air, eat small amounts and chew food thoroughly. Since poor or irregular bowel movements may make gas pains even more intense, establishing good bowel habits is important. Certain foods should be avoided by persons prone to flatulence: fried food, sweet desserts, cucumbers, cabbage, broccoli, beans, parsnips, and corn are often included in lists of gas-forming foods. Again, avoid taking self-prescribed medication. If the above suggestions do not help to prevent or relieve flatulence during pregnancy, a woman should consult her doctor. Persistent cases may require medication.

Constipation

The pressure of the enlarging uterus on the lower portion of the intestine may make elimination of waste difficult. Decreased fluid intakes due to the nausea and/or vomiting of early pregnancy may make constipation a problem during the first trimester. Following the dry-liquid regimen suggested for sufferers of morning sickness will help to ensure adequate fluid intake during the nausea weeks.

Increasing fluid intake, eating plenty of fresh fruits and vegetables, and including adequate bulk in the diet can help a pregnant woman to avoid or cure constipation. Such naturally laxative foods as whole grains with added bran and dried prunes or figs can be used as premeal snacks. Prune juice can be used as the morning fruit juice, provided that citrus fruit or juice or a vegetable high in vitamin C is taken later in the day.

By eating carefully washed, *unpeeled, raw* fruits (apples, pears, peaches, nectarines, grapes, plums) one can add significant amounts of fiber to the diet without adding new foods. Unpeeled tomatoes also add fiber; vegetables such as celery, broccoli, green beans, asparagus, dried peas and beans, rhubarb, cabbage, and sauerkraut are relatively high in fiber content.

Much emphasis is currently being placed on the advantages of adding bran to one's diet. Though the more spectacular claims for bran have not yet been proven, its value as a natural laxative has long been recognized. One-fourth cup of bran, either plain or mixed with a favorite cereal, can become a regular part of breakfast for women with chronic constipation problems. Highly absorbent, bran (fiber) soaks up the liquids of the intestine and increases the bulk of the intestinal waste, enabling fecal contents to stimulate muscular action of the bowel. Bran also promotes the production of certain fatty acids that act as natural laxatives. Unfortunately, bran also tends to bind minerals so that they are eliminated with fecal wastes. Though the use of bran may prove satisfactory for women who have begun bran supplements before conception, women who try the remedy late in pregnancy may experience flatulence and a feeling of fullness if they add the recommended ½ ounce per day all at once. For this reason starting bran consumption in smaller amounts and building up to the needed amount is especially important for pregnant women who wish to take advantage of the natural laxative effects of bran.

Unless ordered by a doctor in extreme cases of constipation, laxatives should be avoided by the pregnant woman. Though a mild laxative is not likely to cause premature labor or other such complications, laxatives tend to bind minerals so that they are eliminated rather than absorbed by the body.

Hemorrhoids

Hemorrhoids during pregnancy are often the result of the pressure exerted by congestion of the pubic veins by the enlarging uterus. They may be aggravated (or even produced) by straining as a result of constipation. Adequate exercise to promote good circulation plus dietary measures recommended for prevention or alleviation of constipation will help to avoid hemorrhoids.

Leg Cramps

Leg cramps—charlie horses—often plague pregnant women. One probable cause of leg cramps is the slowing of blood circulation due to pressure exerted by the growing uterus on the large pelvic blood vessels. Bending the foot upward or pressing it flat against the wall or headboard of the bed may relieve such cramps. Wearing comfortable, moderately low-heeled shoes to prevent putting undue strain on the calf muscles might also help. Certain exercises are especially helpful in preventing and/or relieving leg cramps. Dietary change has sometimes been prescribed for cramps, since they may be caused by an imbalance in the calcium-phosphorus ratio. In times past women have occasionally been advised to eliminate milk from the diet. While drinking excess milk might increase the occurrence of leg cramps, eliminating milk from the diet is ill-advised except in highly unusual cases. Three to four cups (1 quart) of milk or milk foods (i.e., cheese, yogurt, ice cream) are needed to supply adequate protein, calcium, riboflavin, and vitamins A and D. Unless supplements are used to meet these demands, milk should remain in prenatal diets. Since some researchers (Abrams and Aporte, 1958) have maintained that there is insufficient evidence to support the theory that increased milk causes leg cramps, eliminating milk altogether hardly seems warranted. In severe cramping cases physicians have added small quantities of aluminum hydroxide to the daily quart of milk, since this addition will remove some phosphorus from the intestinal tract and help to restore a more desirable calcium-phosphorus ratio.

Anemia

As discussed earlier, two types of anemia, partially due to the large increase in total volume of the maternal blood, are fairly common among pregnant women. If hemoglobin concentrations fall, many factors may be involved, some of which relate to diet. Hemoglobin is a complex iron-protein molecule, requiring the presence of ample supplies of protein, calcium, iron, copper, zinc, folic acid, Vitamin B$_{12}$, and several other vitamins. A malnourished individual is a prime candidate for anemia of this kind.

Even a well-nourished woman may develop anemia during pregnancy—a fact that has led to routine use of iron and folic-acid supplements. Since a woman generally loses .700 to .800 mg of iron during pregnancy, most women need such supplements. Iron-rich foods should also be eaten, since supplementation alone does not ensure against development of anemia.

Megaloblastic anemia, related to folic-acid deficiencies, may occur if too little animal protein, green, leafy vegetables, and other folacin-rich foods are eaten. Nausea and loss of appetite usually occur, both of which tend to compound the problem. Folic-acid supplements plus attention to folacin-rich foods usually prevent anemia of this sort.

Toxemia

Fear of this previously mentioned "disease of theories" has led many women to starve themselves into dangerously low pregnancy weight gains. Current evidence disputes the old theory that weight gain *per se* leads to toxemia, and a pregnant woman should not attempt to prevent toxemia through a self-imposed weight-loss plan.

To ignore the importance of prenatal nutrition and assume that only fate or chance can determine whether or not one's child will be well-born and healthy is to deny facts brought to light by hundreds of studies. Results of these studies clearly indicate that the future of an unborn child may well rest upon the nutritional history and prenatal nutritional status of its mother. Since providing that child with an optimum nutritional environment takes so little effort and pays such large dividends, ignoring that responsibility seems unthinkable.

Part II

Your baby will get off to a fine start on your milk, a nutrition-ally perfect food for the infant. You will want him to build on this good start. The best way to accomplish this is by being a family in which *everyone* has good nutritional habits.

La Leche League International
(The Womanly Art of Breast-Feeding,
2nd edition, Franklin Park, Illinois, 1963)

EXAMINING
POSTPARTUM NUTRITIONAL OPTIONS

The World Health Organization, the American Academy of Pediatrics, the American Public Health Association, and other responsible medical authorities have agreed that breast feeding is the best way to nourish young babies.

Citizen's Committee on Infant Nutrition
(Center for Science in the Public Interest,
Washington, D. C., 1974)

Following the birth of her child a new mother can choose between several nutritional options. All too often she is not even aware that options exist. Some of these options relate to a mother's own nutritional needs; others relate to the needs of her baby.

Maternal Nutritional Options
Except in unusual cases, such as complications of delivery, the American College of Obstetricians and Gynecologists advises that a new mother be given a well-balanced diet, one in which fluids are neither restricted nor markedly increased. The mother who gives birth at a hospital receives such meals for at least the length of her hospital stay. In far too many cases the end of hospitalization means the end of well-balanced meals.

Once her baby has been born, a mother may spend hours seeing that its nutritional needs are met yet fail to allow herself enough time to pause for a good breakfast or an adequate lunch. She may slip into the martyr's role, skipping meals, losing sleep, and generally giving up her own health for that of her child's. Such sacrifice is not only uncalled for but also unfair to the very child whom she believes that she is helping. No baby can be perfectly happy and content with a mother who is hungry, anemic, and tired. Such a mother is likely to shower him with affection one minute, then scream at him the next. If she actually becomes ill, she is even less able to be a good mother.

Some mothers don't assume the martyr's role at all. Having "put up with being fat" for nine months, they are obsessed with the need to crash-diet their way to slimness. Under the pressures of caring for a demanding infant they find starvation dieting easier to accomplish than ever before. They simply forget to eat—or don't manage to find time to eat. Delighted with the thought of rapid weight loss, they fail to consider that a relatively rapid return to preconception weight can be accomplished through safer, less drastic means.

Assuming that the second goal of prenatal weight management has been met, returning to prepregnancy weight is not difficult for most women. That goal involves "keep[ing] the mother from accumulating exessive fat, so that about a month after delivery she can return to within a few pounds of what she weighed before she became pregnant." In view of the bodily changes that occur in the postpartum period this goal is entirely realistic, provided that the mother-to-be has kept her total weight gain reasonably close to the recommended 24 pounds.

To understand how this rapid return to prepregnancy weight is achieved, one must look again at the products of pregnancy given in chapter II.

By subtracting what nature subtracts during delivery and shortly thereafter one can see why such rapid weight loss occurs. At delivery the mother is relieved of the weight of the baby (7.5 pounds), placenta (1 pound) and amniotic fluid (2 pounds), an average total of 10.5 pounds. In addition, she usually has increased excretion in the days immediately following delivery and loses an additional 4 to 5 pounds. These losses, coupled with blood volume adjustments, mean that by the end of the first postpartum week a mother who gained 24 pounds has probably lost 18 to 20 of those pounds.

For the nursing mother the remaining four pounds of "fat reserve" will be rapidly used up as her body calls for extra energy for the manufacture of 30 ounces (600 calories) of milk per day. She has allowed the demands of a growing fetus to dictate her prenatal weight gain, and by allowing her body to meet the demands of a nursing infant she can allow nature to make return to her prepregnant weight a relatively simple matter.

Both the nursing and the nonnursing mother can benefit from a well-structured postpartum-exercise program. Exercise, not drastic calorie cuts, is needed to tone up stretched abdomen and breast muscles, work off fat pockets along the lower back, and lose a few excess pounds. The new mother should ideally discuss her proposed exercise program with her physician, presenting him with exercises that she would like to begin or asking for help in choosing appropriate postpartum exercises. Since she will probably wish to start such a program as soon as possible, she should ask these questions before she leaves the hospital. Unless her own special circumstances dictate otherwise, she can usually proceed with the simplest exercises soon after delivery, adding more strenuous ones at the appropriate time. By the time of her six-week postpartum checkup, she will probably be allowed to resume exercises and activities such as biking, tennis, and swimming.

Following a sound postpartum diet is important to both nursing and nonnursing mothers. Failure to do so jeopardizes not only the mother's health but also that of future children. Immediately following delivery maternal stores are low and should be replenished. For example, the American College of Obstetricians and Gynecologists recommends continuation of iron supplements for at least two or three months postpartum to ensure the replenishing of this vital element.

The new mother who neglects her own nutritional needs will not be her best physical, mental, or emotional self. Furthermore, should she conceive again soon after delivery, she will likely begin the new pregnancy with low, insufficient maternal reserves. After spending nine months in a state of physical exhaustion she will deliver another child, only to return home in her perpetually tired state. While caring for two diaper-aged children she is likely to neglect her own needs still further.

Spacing children at least two or three years apart allows a mother to replenish her body's stores of vital elements, especially iron, before taxing those reserves once more through the stresses of pregnancy. Such spacing, coupled with excellent nutritional practices during the interconceptional years, ensures each child of the best possible nutritional environment during conception and the weeks that immediately follow.

Infant Nutritional Options

"To breast-feed or not to breast-feed" is a relatively new dilemma. Prior to this century choosing *not* to breast-feed an infant was to choose to endanger the life of that child. Sanitation measures were so poor, refrigeration techniques so primitive that bacteria often abounded in the cow's milk fed to a tiny baby. Nature's way was then the only way for a conscientious mother to consider. The gradual move away from breast-feeding came only after sanitation and refrigeration had been improved.

At first only upper-class women bottle-fed, since such feeding was an obvious extra expense for the family. Gradually, as the practice began to become more and more a status symbol, other women made the transition. How often babies have been troubled by intestinal disorders and other illnesses due to the poor handling of bottle-fed milk or formulas is not known.

So great was the rush toward bottle feeding that by the early 1950s breast feeding had become almost a lost art. Young women who wanted to try feeding their infants the natural way had no one to support them in their efforts. With sanitation measures in the United States greatly improved, bottlefeeding seemed safe enough to physicians as well as to mothers. Therefore the medical profession gradually endorsed bottle feeding and made little effort to support those relatively few women who wanted to breast-feed their babies.

In 1956, a group of Illinois women founded La Leche International, a support group dedicated to giving encouragement and assistance to mothers who chose breast feeding. In 1958 they published *The Womanly Art of Breast Feeding,* a guide for nursing mothers. From an initial publication of 17,000 copies the book has had ever-increasing press runs, moving from 10,000 to 50,000 in the decade between 1963 and 1973. The increasing yearly sales of this book, plus the growing membership in La Leche League International, attest to the growing interest in breast feeding.

Who are the breast-feeders of the 1970s? In the United States they are often college-educated, upper-social-class young women, young women who make their own decisions without being unduly swayed by pressures from society. They are slowly influencing other women to turn to breast feeding, but the trend is still a gradual one. In some hospitals as many as 50% to 60% of mothers choose breast over bottle, but in others percentages are much smaller.

Interest in breast-feeding ran high enough at the 1969 White House Conference on Food, Nutrition, and Health to cause Dr. Jean Mayer, Conference Chairman, to attempt a survey of current attitudes toward breast feeding. In 1970 he reported that "It may well be that we are in the midst of a slow change led by the more educated women and community leaders in general." Why are these educated young women deciding to breast-feed their babies? Often they must fight for their right to shun the bottle in favor of the breast, for many physicians and hospital staffs still favor bottle feeding. In hospitals of this type bottle-fed babies can be "managed" with less trouble. Their mothers need not be awakened for nightime feedings. There is no need for busy nurses to assist new mothers in the art of breast feeding.

Fortunately, many physicians are beginning to advise mothers to return to nature's way of infant feeding. Conferences seeking ways to improve the health of children have supported research that has convinced many leading medical personnel that the breast is best. At the 1969 White House Conference on Food, Nutrition, and Health the panel on the family noted that ". . . breast milk is the perfect food for [a baby's] nutritional needs and development; that it is the most natural way to feed babies; and that it provides a protection against infection and allergies that cannot be duplicated."

Physicians who have reeducated themselves in the area of breast feeding are working to change the attitudes and practices of hospital maternity staffs. In hospitals that reflect the trend toward a return to breast feeding, staffs are able to provide new mothers with valuable assistance as they learn to breast-feed their newborns. Of course, the advice and assistance isn't always perfect, for it often comes from nurses who never breast-fed their own infants and who have had years of experience with bottle-feeding mothers and only limited experience with breast-feeding mothers.

Once again, then, a woman who decides to find out what's best for her child and to follow that route may have an uphill climb. She must evaluate the pros-and-cons of breast feeding, make her own decision, then breast- or bottle-feed her child, content that she has made a wise choice. She must realize that breast-feeding is an unadvertised art, since it is not a profit-making activity, whereas bottle-feeding and early feeding of solids are heavily advertised by the many who profit from the sale of formulas and baby foods. She must look at the facts, evaluate the benefits, then make her own decision.

Fears About Breast Feeding

Many women, brought up in homes in which bottle-feeding was the norm, have very real fears about breast feeding. They may refuse to consider it simply because they have let these fears rule their thinking. By taking an honest look at those fears they may find that they have worried needlessly.

The breast has been removed from the nursery and placed in the master bedroom, becoming a symbol of sexual gratification instead of a means of infant nutrition. Many young women, viewing the breast as sexual, seem repulsed by the idea of using the breast to meet a baby's needs. There need be no either-or decision on this point. Women who nurse their babies report no declining interest in sexual pleasure. Provided that their husbands can be educated to the advantages of breast feeding, there seems to be no significant modification of love-making techniques. Many fear drastic changes in breast appearance after nursing. While there are no definitive research statistics to disprove this fear, many studies suggest that breast changes are usually the result of pregnancy, not of lactation.

The working mother's fears about breast feeding are legitimate ones. Obviously a mother who is able to be at home all day with her baby finds nursing that baby a relatively easy task. However, as of March 1973, only 29.4% of mothers with children under age three were in the working force. Of that number an even smaller percentage had babies under six months of age. Based on these figures, over three-quarters of American women could nurse their babies for at least six months without giving up their jobs in order to do so. Even those who must return to work soon after the baby's birth can choose to breast-feed. Some employers offer short nursing breaks in lieu of long lunch hours. Others are even providing day-care facilities, which mean that a mother is always fairly close to her child, ready to meet his needs. Other mothers leave bottles of formula for a sitter to feed to the baby, and still others hand-express milk or use a pump to fill bottles for their infants. Working and breast feeding are not mutually exclusive activities. If a mother wants to nurse her child, she can do so, even if she must work outside the home.

Many women claim that they don't know how to breast-feed. This was a legitimate cry for a good many years, since breast-feeding was diminishing so rapidly that supportive advice was not readily available. With the founding of La Leche League International and the changing of physicians' attitudes, new mothers can usually find good literature and obtain sound guidance if they choose to breast-feed.

With breast cancer no longer a hush-hush disease, women are attempting to learn all they can about prevention and early detection of this often fatal disease. Many fear that nursing will cause cancer, but current research indicates that mothers who breast-feed their babies for at least nine months may be less susceptible to cancer than nonnursing mothers. The hormonal changes that are associated with prolonged lactation may offer protection against breast cancer. These hormonal changes, similar to those seen in women who have "stairstep babies," seem to discourage the development of cancer. In short, while there is no evidence to support the rumor that breast feeding *causes* breast cancer, there is some evidence to suggest that breast feeding may inhibit its development. Nursing does not, of course, rule out the possibility of cancer. Even the woman who nurses her children for long periods of time may under certain circumstances develop breast cancer. All women should continue to watch for early signs of this disease.

Nursing mothers have often been warned against eating certain foods that might cause discomfort to the baby. If the baby has colic, Grandmother insists that the new mother should avoid chocolate, while Auntie is just as sure that yesterday's Mexican food caused the problem. In reality baby may be upset for reasons completely unrelated to mother's diet. La Leche League International, the largest organization of breast-feeding women, suggests that a nursing mother should not feel that baby's every gas pain is caused by something that she ate. A nervous, guilt-ridden mother may even help to bring on a case of colic by transferring to the nursing baby her own anxieties about the food that she has eaten. A mother who begins a nursing experience with positive attitudes about all foods is more likely to enjoy that experience than a mother who anticipates trouble from the start. The nursing mother should refuse the martyr's role. Instead she should assume that a normal, well-balanced diet will be satisfactory for the baby, omitting certain foods only if she is positive that they are causing trouble.

No scientific method of isolating potential trouble-making foods has as yet been devised. Too many variables exist to make a conclusive study of such matters possible. Digestive systems vary from mother to mother and from baby to baby. Highly spiced chili that causes heartburn in one woman may be consumed without ill effects by another. Conversely, the first mother's baby might show no signs of distress after a secondhand chili meal; the second mother's child might scream as if in protest. How can one be sure that the chili caused baby's distress? Only by ruling out every other possible cause (a slight cold, earache, loss of sleep) *and*, if chili happens to be one of her favorite foods, trying two or three more chili meals to see whether similar reactions occur, can she began to say with certainty that eating chili bothers the baby. Even then her own fears that colic might occur could be causing more gastric distress to the baby then does the chili.

A verbal survey of any group of nursing mothers usually yields a wide variety of foods avoided for baby's sake. The foods that are named most often may, indeed, *be* colic-causers. On the other hand, they may be foods that the mothers have been led to *believe* would cause colic. For whatever reasons some foods do continue to be mentioned more than others. Many mothers report problems after eating cabbage (cooked or raw), broccoli, baked beans, onions, fried foods, chocolate, cantaloupe, watermelon, and spicy foods—while others do not. Some women indicate that many foods that seemed to cause colic in a newborn had no adverse effect after the baby was three to four months old.

Since the state of *two* bodies must be considered in evaluating the influence of maternal diet on an infant's digestive system, the probability is great that dietary intolerance for mother and baby is a matter of individual differences. There is no evidence to indicate that *all* nursing mothers should avoid eating certain foods. It's a matter of individual differences.

In the belief that each nursing mother must decide for herself which, if any, foods she should avoid for baby's sake, no effort was made to exclude certain dishes from menu plans for the lactating mother. Baked beans, spicy barbeques and other traditionally off-limits foods can probably be enjoyed by most mothers with no ill effects on baby, unless they are eaten in unusually large quantities or under adverse circumstances.

Facts About Breast Feeding
The increasing interest in breast feeding can probably be attributed to the growing realization that it has advantages over bottle feeding that had heretofore not been realized. For both mother and baby nursing offers unique advantages, most of which cannot be duplicated by even the most advanced formula. The Committee on Nutrition of the American Academy of Pediatrics reported that: "Infants grow most rapidly during the first 4 to 6 months of life. Nutrient requirements are most critical in this period, during which nutritional deficiencies can have lasting effects on growth and development . . . Breast milk has not been improved upon as a reference standard."

Ironically, while breast milk has been used as a reference standard against which to measure infant formulas based on cow's milk and soy protein, it has not been seriously reconsidered as the *ideal formula* until recent years. Growing numbers of pediatricians are endorsing breast feeding after seeing the difference that it can make in their own patients and reading statistics that indicate the difference that it can make in others. Faced with growing evidence that breast is best, they have begun to encourage mothers who want to adopt the natural way of infant feeding.

Tables comparing human milk with cow's milk and/or cow's-milk formulas show the extent to which formula-makers have tried to imitate the composition of human milk. While vitamin and mineral supplements have helped to bring the imitation milks closer to the original, some basic differences still exist.

Human milk is fairly low in casein yet high in lactalbumin. Cow's milk is high in casein and low in lactalbumin. Since lactalbumin is considered the optimum protein for infant growth and casein is a relatively hard-to-digest protein, the advantages of human milk should be obvious. Calves grow three times as fast as babies, and cow's milk is ideally suited to accomplish this rapid growth. The human child has different patterns of development and needs different nutrients to promote optimum growth. Human milk is ideally suited to meet those needs.

A closer look at the composition of human milk should help to clarify this point of view. Calories for cow's milk and human milk are about equal—67 per 100 milligrams. Protein is more abundant in cow's milk, but the protein in human milk is easier to digest and thus more efficiently utilized. The decreased amount of casein means that smaller, softer, more easily digested curds form in the stomach. Fat content of cow's milk and human milk is almost the same, but human milk is high in polyunsaturated fats and essential fatty acids. It is also high in lipase, an enzyme that enhances the availablity of essential fatty acids. Human milk contains more cholesterol than does cow's milk. Cholesterol is vital to the synthesis of bile acids and male and female sex hormones, and recent studies indicate that cholesterol in an infant's diet can spur the development of natural regulatory mechanisms for cholesterol metabolism.

This last factor is of great importance to citizens of a nation plagued by heart disease, which is thought to be related to abnormally high serum-cholesterol levels. Increasing evidence seems to support the theory that infants may need a moderate amount of dietary cholesterol in order to establish mechanisms for proper metabolism of cholesterol in later life. Low-cholesterol infant formulas, once thought desirable, may actually be contributing to atheromatous-arteriosclerosis problems in later life.

Sodium content of cow's milk is far greater than that of human milk (25 to 30 milligrams per liter vs 7 milligrams per liter). Most infant formulas fall somewhere between the two extremes. Since there is evidence that excessive salt intakes may lead to high blood pressure at an early adult age in persons predisposed to hypertension, the lower sodium content of breast milk seems highly desirable.

Mineral content of human milk differs significantly from that of cow's milk. The higher calcium: phosphorus ratio of breast milk encourages more total absorption of calcium. Convulsions during the first two weeks of life have been traced to low-calcium, elevated-phosphorus levels in the blood of babies fed a cow's-milk formula. The much larger phosphorus content of cow's milk (96% versus 15% in human milk) has been linked to such problems as neonatal hypoparathyroidism. Increased incidence of hypocalcemia (13.3% in cow's-milk-formula babies versus 0% for breast-milk babies) has also been noted.

Infant formulas fortified with iron provide more iron than does breast milk, but if the mother used an iron supplement during pregnancy, the newborn's iron stores should be sufficient for his first few months of life. If a mother did not use prenatal iron supplements, a breast-fed infant may need iron supplementation. Since cow's milk alone is also low in iron, the same rule applies to babies fed cow's milk or cow's-milk formulas that have not been fortified with iron.

Vitamin content of human milk seems perfectly suited to meet an infant's needs except for Vitamin D. In cold or smoggy climates in which a baby gets minimum exposure to sunlight and therefore has limited opportunity to synthesize adequate amounts of Vitamin D, supplementation may be advised. In most other cases human milk is used as the reference standard for the vitamin content of man-made formulas based on cow's milk and/or soy protein.

Since technology has enabled formula manufacturers to approximate the nutrient composition of human milk, why have leading authorities begun to insist that breast milk must still be considered the ideal food? The World Health Organization, the American Academy of Pediatrics, and the American Public Health Association are a few of the many responsible medical authorities who have agreed that breast feeding is the best way to nourish young babies. Their conclusion is based on more than a comparison of the nutritional content of breast milk and infant formulas.

Newborns enter life with certain protective antibodies at work, antibodies gained from the mother during the prenatal months. In the most natural birth setting the mother allows the infant to nurse at her breast within minutes after birth, and colostrum, the yellowish fluid that he receives in this early nursing experience, gives him additional immunity against harmful bacteria. Leukocytes in colstrum may prevent necrotizing enterocolitis, an often deadly infection common to newborns who have undergone blood transfusions. High concentrations of certain lymphocyles in breast milk can line part of the baby's intestinal tract and give protection against harmful bacteria, protection that the baby does not receive to a significant degree in the prenatal environment.

If the mother has an infection, her colostrum provides the baby with antibodies against that infection. Since the baby is likely to encounter certain harmful bacteria during its trip through the birth canal, such antibodies can prove invaluable in combating those bacteria. Even in high-risk environments 100%-breast-fed babies are often able to avoid shigella and certain salmonellas, including typhoid fever.

Human milk contains a group of complex starches that promotes the growth of certain intestinal bacteria that produce an acid environment unfriendly to the growth of disease-causing microorganisms. No other infant formula can offer the unique immunological advantages of breast milk. According to the Center for Science in the Public Interest, "The combined effect of the anti-infective factors suggests that human milk is superior to any other milk for infants".

One further immunological point should be made. Totally breast-fed infants are less likely to develop cow's-milk allergy, the most common allergy of infancy. Ten percent of American infants on formulas use soy-protein-base formulas. These infants have displayed allergic reactions to cow's milk. Withholding cow's milk for the first three months of life may minimize chances of allergic reactions. In families with a history of allergies mothers are being strongly encouraged to breast-feed their babies. In summary, John W. Gerrard's comment in *Pediatrics,* December 1974, is appropriate: "We now know that breastfeeding insures a smooth transition for the baby from being entirely dependent on his mother for both his nutritional and immunologic requirements to being completely independent. It is this new awareness of the limitations of formula feeding . . . that makes us have second thoughts on breast-feeding."

One of the most interesting theories being explored by those interested in breast feeding involves infant appetite control. While properly working adult body mechanisms convey a feeling of fullness when an adequate number of calories has been consumed, the infant's appetite-control apparatus apparently responds to volume, not to caloric intake. According to one British researcher breast milk is ideally suited to this method of appetite control, because it is not consistently high in calories. At the beginning of a feeding the milk is thin. It then becomes creamy, returns to thin, then back to creamy. Thus the baby's thirst can be satified by relatively large volumes of breast milk, all of which is not necessarily high in calories.

Both mother and baby can benefit from the close contact essential to breast feeding. According to a recent work on maternal-infant bonding, touch is an important element in establishing a firm bond. Suckling a child enhances the relationship. The hormone prolactin is considered a love hormone in birds. There is speculation that the human mother's attachment to her infant may be enhanced by increased prolactin secretion. This may be nature's way of helping to ensure survival of the newborn.

Bonding is further enhanced by the infant's ability to distinguish its mother's milk from the milk of other mothers by its odor. The tiny child can make this distinction as early as the fifth day. For many mothers there is a strong sense of pride and well-being associated with being the chief provider of the baby's needs. Most nursing mothers enjoy the intimate physical contact that breast feeding allows, and there is increasingly strong evidence to support the idea that the baby gains a sense of security from this close, one-to-one relationship.

Other advantages of breast feeding include oxytocin production. The stimulation of the mother's breast during nursing signals release of oxytocin, a powerful hormone that causes uterine contractions and helps the uterus to return to its prepregnancy size. These contractions may also help to prevent postpartum hemorrhaging.

The convenience of breast-feeding is often overlooked by mothers-to-be who fear that they will be tied down by a nursing baby. Wherever mother is, there is also a sterile, nutritious food supply, ready and at the perfect temperature. Night feedings are ready in seconds, since there is no bottle to be heated. The *economy* of breast feeding may become an increasingly important factor in our overpopulated world. The mother's daily need for extra calories, protein, and calcium can be met by adding to her normal diet a peanut butter-and-jelly sandwich and a glass of milk at a cost of less than half a dollar. The formula necessary to feed a child costs considerably more and offers considerably less than the breast milk that the mother can so easily produce.

Finally, breast feeding can provide an easy method of losing a few excess pounds. Provided that a woman follows the dietary recommendations given within this guide, she can meet her own needs and those of her baby and still whittle away a few pounds. Nursing should never be an excuse for obesity. Instead it might well open the door to slimness.

In summary, all current medical evidence seems to support breast feeding as the ideal way to nurture an infant. Of course, when the art of breast feeding becomes a fetish or an end in itself, an infant may suffer. For example, infants limited to breast milk alone for periods beyond nine months tend to develop marked deficiency symptoms. The important thing is to seek the *best* nutritional experience for a newborn, and apparently breast *is* best, at least for the first three to six months of life. As Dr. Jean Mayer has noted: "Natural nursing is a foolproof method which can be duplicated only by intelligent, constantly careful, clinically guided—and costlier—artificial feeding. Under less than ideal conditions, morbidity and mortality are consistently greater in artificially fed infants than in breast-fed."

After examining the postpartum nutritional options open to her, the new mother must decide whether breast feeding or bottle feeding seems best suited to her particular situation. No matter how potentially advantageous breast feeding is for babies, a mother who knows that she cannot feel comfortable in a nursing role should probably not take on such a role. After all, a baby senses adult emotions too well to receive optimum benefits from a feeding method for which his mother feels strong dislike.

Whether a mother chooses breast or formula as a means of nourishing her infant, she must still be aware of her obligation to meet her own nutritional needs. The following two chapters are addressed to the postpartum needs of the nursing and nonnursing mother. Once the lactating mother has weaned her child, she may find the latter chapter helpful as she adjusts her caloric load to postlactation levels.

UNDERSTANDING AND MEETING THE NUTRITIONAL NEEDS OF THE NURSING MOTHER

> The lactating mother requires more dietary additions than does the pregnant woman.
>
> Sue Rodwell Williams
> *(Nutrition and Diet Therapy,*
> C. V. Mosby Company, St. Louis, 1969)

White House Conference on Food, Nutrition, and Health stated in its sixth recommendation that "Thought must be given to the fact that a nursing mother must have a good diet, in addition to enough sleep and relaxation, or she will not produce milk of . . . sufficient quality." The quotation states facts that should be obvious. After all, breast milk must be produced by the mother, and production of milk requires energy. Unfortunately, many young mothers tend to neglect their own nutritional needs, even while expressing great concern for the needs of their new babies. In cases in which breast feeding gets off to a strong start, the baby may not suffer appreciably from his mother's poor diet, even though his mother may develop significant deficiency symptoms. In other cases the poor quality of a mother's postpartum diet may doom any attempts at breast feeding.

Milk Quantity

If caloric intakes are insufficient to provide for the manufacture of breast milk, milk production will fall below optimum levels. Milk quantity is definitely related to maternal caloric intake. As Adelle Davis has noted in *Let's Have Healthy Children:*

> "As a nursing mother doing your own housework and perhaps caring for other children, your calorie requirement is comparable to that of a day laborer. Getting too few calories can decrease your milk supply and cause both your dietary protein and body protein to be wastefully used as calories. The fact that your requirement for calories is high, however, should not be used as an excuse for eating junk food. Let everything you eat build health."

Caloric intakes of nursing women should be even greater than those for pregnant women, for the rapidly growing infant's needs are even greater than those of the fetus. An autonomous creature, the newborn must now regulate his own body temperature, a process requiring extra energy. He is also freer to move about than he was within the confines of the womb. His tissue metabolism is less efficient now than during his intrauterine days, and he is no longer being fed by the highly efficient placental-transfer system. Instead he is receiving milk produced by his mother's body, the best possible food for him at this age, yet a food for which he must work. During his mother's last trimester of pregnancy he was growing rapidly and demanding many calories, but she was moving more slowly than usual, acutely conscious of his ever-increasing size and weight. She ate well for the sake of her growing child. Suddenly her days of slow movement are over. She must be in at least three different places at once. She does all that she did before the child's arrival and also manages to meet his demands. Somehow she has lost sight of the fact that she is now feeding two separate organisms, a task that requires quality calories in sufficient quantity to meet her own needs and those of her child.

Anxious to lose weight quickly and ignorant of the nutritional needs of lactation, she tries to carry a tremendous physical load without adequate energy intake. If she succeeds in nursing her child, it may be at great cost to her own health. More often she soon gives up the endeavor, convinced that she just hasn't got what it takes to breast-feed a child. And, if her diet is inadequate, she dosen't have what it takes, for breast feeding requires energy. Her grandmother had the necessary energy because she believed the old "eating for two" adage and because she wasn't so obsessed with slimness that she neglected to eat well during her nursing months.

Today's educated young woman has gone full circle, reversing the trend away from breast feeding and seeking the benefits that nursing can bring to mother and child. All too often she has proceeded by trial and error in the area of nutrition, unsure which advice should be taken seriously and unable to determine herself the number of extra calories that nursing requires. Until the past few years leading authorities recommended 1,000 extra calories per day. Since human milk production averages 30 ounces (850 ml) per day and contains 20 calories per ounce, the average nursing mother daily manufactures milk containing 600 calories. Assuming, as authorities once did, that maternal energy is converted to milk energy with about 60% efficiency, production of 600 calories of milk would require about 1,000 extra calories per day. However, in 1970 research teams discovered that milk production was a more efficient process than had been assumed. This group asserted that maternal energy is converted to milk energy with about 80% efficiency. Under this assumption production of 600 calories of breast milk would require maternal intakes of approximately 750 additional calories.

Still another factor must be considered in setting caloric requirements. Women who gain the recommended number of pounds (24 to 27) have body fat stored as a nursing reserve to help them through the first months of lactation. This 2- to 4-kg (4- to 8-pound) reserve should provide about 200 to 300 kcal/ day during a lactation period of about 100 days, thus meeting one-third of the caloric cost of average milk production per day. During that first 100 days a nursing mother should add an extra 500 calories to her nonpregnant diet to meet the remaining two-thirds of the milk-production energy costs. This is only a 200-calorie increase over the prenatal diet that she has followed for the past few months. Adding only 500 extra calories per day (200 above prenatal levels) allows fat deposits to be used up as nature intended. Adding double that amount would probably mean that those deposits would stay—in the form of unsightly bulges. Once lactation has been well-established (beyond the third month), a mother may need to begin adding snacks to make up for the 200 to

300 calories per day that her postpartum fat reserves are no longer supplying. The added 200 to 300 calories (a total of 750 to 800 per day) should in theory enable a mother to nurse yet maintain a steady weight. The new mother who wishes to gain a few pounds will need to be especially careful not to omit needed calories, lest she find that she is losing, not gaining. The new mother who wants to lose a few pounds can do so safely and easily by leaving her extra-calorie load at the 500 mark once the first three months of lactation have passed. She may even be able to lower that number to 400 and still provide ample calories for her own needs, relying for some of her energy on the calories that will be lost as body fat is utilized for milk production. As long as she maintains a well-balanced diet, rich in the nutrients essential to her own health and necessary for adequate milk production, she can lose weight without sacrificing her health or that of her nursing child. As Karen Pryor writes in *Nursing Your Baby:*

"Part of enjoying life in these first six weeks [of nursing] is eating heartily and well. This is not the time to "diet"; lactation is the best "diet" there is, anyway. A few months or a year of giving milk can strip unnecessary weight from you without the slightest effort on your part. Some mothers think that the most enjoyable thing about lactation is that for a few happy months they can dive into meals with gusto, eating cream on the cereal and two helpings of everything, and never gain a pound."

ENERGY RECOMMENDATIONS DURING LACTATION

Age (years)	Weight (kg)	(lbs)	Height (cm)	(in)	Nonpregnant Nonlactating Energy Requirements (kcal/day)		Energy for Lactation (kcal/day)		Lactation Energy Requirements (kcal/day)
11-14	44	97	155	62	2400	+	500	=	2900
15-18	54	119	162	65	2100	+	500	=	2600
19-22	58	128	162	65	2100	+	500	=	2600
23-50	58	128	162	65	2000	+	500	=	2500

The above energy (calorie) figures are based on an average milk prodution of 600 calories per day, the amount of milk usually manufactured by a woman who is exclusively breast feeding one child. The mother of twins would need more calories. Conversely, the working woman who gives only a morning and evening feeding and relies on formula feedings throughout the day would not produce 600 calories of milk per day and would consequently not need as many extra calories to accomplish her milk production.

As a mother begins to add solid foods to baby's diet, baby may nurse less frequently. As the baby grows more interested in taking milk or other liquids in a bottle or cup and less interested in the breast, he may nurse only a few times a day. During the last weeks or months of the nursing period the baby may nurse only once a day. Since baby-led weaning is such a gradual process, a mother may forget to wean herself! Moving from the 500 or more additional calories required at peak nursing time to her weight-maintenance calorie level is also easier if it is done gradually. In most cases, a woman's appetite diminishes as nursing frequency decreases. In other cases appetite may not prove a reliable guide. When nursing is reduced by one-fourth, caloric intake is reduced by one-fourth. When it is reduced by one-third, intake is reduced by one-third and so on.

Studies involving lactating women indicate that increasing fluids has no significant effect on breast milk supply. Nonetheless, a nursing mother's own body may require additional fluids to make up for those lost in the milk that she is producing.

If fluid intakes are low, urine becomes highly concentrated, and bowel movements may be dry and hard to pass. To offset such effects, a mother can drink extra fluids whenever she feels thirsty. If she doesn't feel thirsty but does feel that fluid intake should be raised, she can remind herself to take a drink of water whenever she nurses the baby. She may choose to take most of her fruit exchanges in juice form.

The nursing mother who receives calories, protein, vitamins, and minerals in the amounts recommended by the food and nutrition board of the National Research Council will be safeguarding her own health and producing sufficient quantities of high-quality milk to meet the needs of her growing child.

Milk Quality

Milk quality is generally not greatly affected by the mother's nutritional status. As long as she is getting enough calories to allow her to produce milk, the quality of that milk remains fairly constant. If her calorie level falls too low, milk production all but ceases, yet the quality of milk produced in small amounts approximates the quality of milk produced in larger amounts from abundant calories. One probable exception is important. Though protein, carbohydrate, and fat contents of milk are not significantly altered by maternal diet, vitamin levels in the milk may be appreciably lowered if the mother's diet is not well-balanced.

At what cost does milk quality remain fairly consistent even if caloric intakes are low enough to cause decreases in milk quantity? Can "empty" calories be consumed without adversely affecting milk quality? How is milk quality maintained under such conditions? The mother's body provides needed nutrients for the production of high-quality milk as long as her own reserves last. A malnourished mother will gradually begin to show deficiency symptoms. If her child is receiving only breast milk and the volume of milk is too low to meet that child's needs, he too will suffer. To protect her own health, a mother should make sure that she consumes well-balanced meals and quality snacks, not just empty calories. Though there are many unanswered questions concerning maternal nutrition during lactation the RDA has set standards for protein, vitamin, and mineral intakes that should be high enough to ensure protection of the health of both mother and child.

Approximately 2 grams of high-quality dietary protein are needed to produce 1 gram of milk protein. Since each day's milk production contains 8 to 10 grams of protein, at least 20 extra grams of protein per day are needed by a lactating woman. The lactating mother whose prenatal diet followed the guidelines given earlier in this book needs to add only 10 additional grams to her prenatal diet, 8 of which can be obtained by adding 8 ounces of milk to her daily diet plan.

RECOMMENDED DAILY DIETARY ALLOWANCES FOR PROTEIN, VITAMINS AND MINERALS

	Nonpregnant, Nonlactating Women				All Lactating Women
AGE (years)	11-14	15-18	19-22	23-50	The + sign indicates
WEIGHT (g)	44	54	58	58	that the specific
WEIGHT (lbs)	97	119	128	128	number following it
HEIGHT (cm)	155	162	162	162	must be added to
HEIGHT (ft.)	5'2"	5'5"	5'5"	5'5"	the daily allowance
					for whichever age,
					weight and height
					concerns you.
PROTEIN	44	48	46	46	+20
FAT-SOLUBLE VITAMINS					
A Activity (RE)	800	800	800	800	1200
A Activity (IU)	4000	4000	4000	4000	6000
D (IU)	400	400	400	—	400
E Activity (IU)	12	12	12	12	15
WATER-SOLUBLE VITAMINS					
C Ascorbic Acid (mg)	45	45	45	45	80
B_9 Folic Acid (mg)	.400	.400	.400	.400	.600
B_5 Niacin (mg)	16	14	14	13	+4
B_2 Riboflavin (mg)	1.3	1.4	1.4	1.2	+0.5
B_1 Thiamin (mg)	1.2	1.1	1.1	1.0	+0.3
B_6 Pyridoxine (mg)	1.6	2.0	2.0	2.0	2.5
B_{12} Cobalamin (mg)	.003	.003	.003	.003	.004
MINERALS					
Calcium (mg)	1200	1200	800	800	1200
Phosphorus (mg)	1200	1200	800	800	1200
Iodine (mg)	.115	.115	.100	.100	.150
Iron (mg)	18	18	18	18	18
Magnesium (mg)	300	300	300	300	450
Zinc (mg)	15	15	15	15	25

As in the case of calories, the amount of extra protein needed will depend on the amount of milk being produced. As the baby is weaned. the mother can lower protein intakes accordingly. A low-protein diet will eventually curtail milk production but will not have very much effect on milk composition. Since the nitrogen content of human milk is not largely protein nitrogen, larger maternal intakes of protein nitrogen do little for the quality of human milk protein.

The nursing mother's diet should provide her with sufficient amounts of key vitamins to meet her own needs plus those of the baby whom she is feeding. Reviewing the prenatal discussion of fat- and water-soluble vitamins should serve as a reminder of the best food sources for each of these vitamins. The Daily Meal Pattern Chart for Lactating Mothers (in this chapter) allows for these increased needs.

In most cases the extent to which the vitamin content of a mother's diet can influence the vitamin content of the milk that she produces is still not known. Recommended daily dietary vitamin allowances for lactating women are calculated in most cases according to the amount of each vitamin present in the breast milk.

Vitamin A is secreted in human milk, and the lactating mother needs an additional 2,000 IU to compensate for the amount that she loses in milk each day. Vitamin D, though necessary for proper absorption of calcium, satisfactory growth rate, and normal mineralization of bone in infants, is not present in breast milk in significant amounts. Even if the mother takes vitamin-D supplements to bring her own intake above the recommended level of 400 IU per day, she cannot significantly raise the vitamin-D content of her breast milk. For this reason the recommended daily dietary allowance for the lactating mother is 400 IU, the amount thought necessary to meet the mother's own needs during the increased activity associated with milk production. Most women receive vitamin D in fortified milk. If a woman gets a lot of sunshine, she probably will not need a vitamin-D supplement. Under certain circumstances physicians may recommend vitamin D tablets (400 IU per day) to avoid the risk of poor calcium absorption at a time when a woman is taking in larger amounts of calcium in order to prevent demineralization of her own bones and teeth during the months when milk production demands much calcium from her body. Since this vitamin is toxic in large amounts, it should be used only under medical supervision.

The baby's needs for vitamin D should not be forgotten. Rickets have occurred in breast-fed infants, though the calcium:phosphorus ratio in human milk seems to make its incidence relatively rare. If babies are exposed to at least one-half hour of sunshine each day, they can probably synthesize enough of this vitamin to meet their needs. However, in cold or smoggy climates adequate exposure to sunlight may be extremely difficult. When in doubt, a woman should ask her pediatrician to recommend a vitamin-D supplement.

A word of caution is needed concerning the use of vitamins for infants. As the prenatal discussion of these vitamins indicated, large doses of vitamins A and D can be toxic. For a child under three months of age ingesting an entire bottle (approximately 50 ml) of vitamin A-and-D preparation could prove fatal. Such preparations should be kept out of reach of toddlers or older children who might decide to make a game of giving vitamins to baby.

Twice as much vitamin E is contained in human milk as in cow's milk. To make up for the two to five IU per liter secreted in breast milk, three IU of this vitamin should be added to the mother's daily diet. Vitamin-K deficiency has been noted in newborn infants, and it may lead to hemorrhaging. Breast milk does not contain sufficient amounts of vitamin K to offset such hemorrhaging, but increasing the amount of vitamin-K-rich foods in the maternal diet does not significantly increase the amount of the vitamin in breast milk. Hemorrhage can be offset or prevented in newborns by giving the baby injections of synthetic vitamin K. Since extreme deficiency is rare and is present only during the first days of life, a nursing mother should not worry unduly about low vitamin-K levels of human milk. Maternal megadoses of the vitamin are not recommended as means of raising the vitamin-K content of milk. Such doses would probably prove ineffective and might be dangerous to the mother.

The recommended daily dietary allowances for water-soluble vitamins can be met by following the Daily Meal Pattern Chart for Lactating Mothers.

If a mother maintains an adequate diet, her milk will contain approximately 35 mg of vitamin C for every 850 ml produced. To help the lactating woman meet this increased demand for vitamin C, 80 mg has been set as the recommended daily dietary allowance. This 20 mg increase over the diet of a pregnant woman can be met by including two or more fair sources of vitamin C in each day's diet or by consuming at least six ounces of orange juice each day.

Folic-acid (B9) requirements for the lactating woman, 200 mg lower than during pregnancy, are still 200 mg higher than those of the nonpregnant, nonlactating female. Some cases of megaloblastic anemia of infancy have been attributed to dietary folic-acid deficiency. In one such case megaloblastic anemia in a three-month-old nursing infant was successfully treated by giving folic-acid supplements to the mother. The average nursing mother secretes approximately .05 mg of folic acid per day in her milk. Since the absorption efficiency of folic acid is about 25%, an additional .200 mg per day should be added to the mother's diet. The Meal Pattern Chart for Lactating Mothers (in this chapter) should enable her to meet or exceed the recommended folic acid allowance.

Niacin (B5) requirements are based on calorie intakes. Since a lactating woman is advised to consume 500 extra calories per day, 4 mg of niacin should be added to her daily diet.

Riboflavin (B2) requirements during lactation are assumed to increase by an amount equal to that secreted daily in the milk. Assuming that utilization efficiency of additional riboflavin is only about 70%, the RDA suggests that a lactating woman add 0.5 mg of this vitamin to her diet each day.

While roboflavin deficiency in the nursing infant or lactating mother is fairly rare, thiamin deficiency has been noted in breast-fed infants whose mothers received insufficient quantities of that vitamin. The existence of infantile beriberi in breast-fed babies seems to indicate that maternal thiamin intake can affect the thiamin level of breast milk. Since 0.1 to 0.2 mg of thiamin are secreted in the daily milk supply, the lactating woman should have additional daily intakes of this vitamin. Increasing daily thaimin intake by 0.3 mg has been recommended.

Pyridoxine (B6) is an important vitamin for both infant and mother. The average mother's milk contains 0.01 to 0.02 mg/liter in the first days of lactation and about 0.2 mg/liter thereafter. The amount of pyridoxine secreted in milk seems to be affected by maternal diet. Since deficiency symptoms have been noted in nursing babies whose mother's milk contained only 0.06 to 0.08 mg/liter, mothers should be careful to follow recommended daily dietary allowances of 2.5 mg for pyridoxine.

Cobalamin (B12) content of human milk per day is minuscule but vital. If a mother's own serum-B$_{12}$ levels are adequate, her milk contains adequate amounts of this vitamin to meet her baby's needs. If the mother's serum levels are not adequate, her baby may show B$_{12}$-deficiency symptoms. To keep the lactating woman's B$_{12}$ levels adequate, the RDA for cobalamin has been set at .004 mg per day.

The diet of the nursing mother must meet her ordinary mineral needs plus those special needs imposed by the stresses of lactation. The Daily Meal Pattern Chart for Lactating Mothers (at the end of this chapter) is designed to ensure adequate mineral intakes during lactation. The discussion that follows should help a nursing mother to understand why certain mineral requirements are increased.

Calcium, a mineral of vital importance to a baby's growth, is secreted in mother's milk at the rate of 250 to 300 mg per day. Mothers with unusually high milk production may secrete as much as 1 g per day. Based on the average figures, the National Research Council's Food and Nutrition Board has recommended a daily dietary intake of 1,200 mg of calcium. Mothers of twins and other mothers who produce unusually large quantities of milk may need even more of this mineral. If a nursing mother fails to consume enough calcium to meet her own needs plus the demands of milk production, her body begins to give up its own calcium supply to allow milk quality to remain constant. Since this calcium must be taken from the bones of the mother, her bones may become bendy. If the reduced calcium level of the mother continues long enough, permanent bone deformities may result. Elevating the calcium level of the mother's diet does little to elevate the calcium of breast milk, but simultaneous additions of vitamin D and calcium have been known to increase the calcium content of milk by as much as 25%. Trying to raise calcium content of human milk above the normal range is not desirable, since too much calcium can cause hypercalcemia in susceptible babies. Cow's milk has a much higher calcium content than does breast milk, and sensitive babies on a cow's milk formula have developed hypercalcemia. A nursing mother who consumes the recommended amounts of calcium (1,200 mg per day) should be able to protect her own body from calcium loss and to produce milk with calcium content at optimum levels. One quart of milk can provide the 1,200 mg, but since a mother may unknowingly fall into the high-milk-production category, an additional eight ounces of milk or an equivalent milk product is usually advised for nursing mothers. Accordingly, the Daily Meal Pattern Chart for Lactating Mothers is based on five servings of milk or milk products.

Phosphorus, another mineral necessary for a baby's growth and development, is less prevalent in breast milk than in cow's milk. The calcium:phosphorus ratio of breast milk is considered the optimum ratio for infants. The nursing mother's daily dietary allowance for phosphorus, equal to that for calcium (1,200 mg), is met by including four to five servings of milk in each day's meals and/or snacks.

The amount of magnesium secreted in the milk of well-nourished mothers seems adequate to meet the needs of nursing infants. The RDA for magnesium has been set at 450 mg per day to keep the mother's own levels adequate during her months of milk production.

Sodium and potassium levels of breast milk, lower than those of cow's milk, meet the infant's needs without overworking his kidneys. Sodium and potassium contents of breast milk are apparently not greatly influenced by maternal diet. The low-sodium advantage of breast feeding is lessened, of course, by early introduction of commercial baby foods which are high in salt.

Iron stores of the nursing mother, like those of the nonnursing mother, should be replenished during the postpartum period. The American College of Obstetricians and Gynecologists recommends continuing prenatal iron supplements for two to three months postpartum to allow for replacement of maternal stores lost during pregnancy. Iron content of human milk is higher than that of cow's milk, but neither milk contains enough iron to meet a baby's needs beyond six months of age. Since most babies are introduced to solids around the middle of the first year, their iron needs are probably met through this means. Before six months of age the baby's iron stores, a legacy from prenatal days, are ample for his needs. Of course, if a mother suffered from severe iron-deficiency anemia during the latter months of her pregnancy, her baby's iron stores might not be able to meet his needs. In such a case a physician might prescribe iron supplements. Since such supplements may be harsh on a baby's digestive system, they should not be given unless a physicians feels that they are absolutely necessary to prevent anemia. Maternal diet apparently has very little influence on the iron content of human milk. Therefore the RDA for nursing mothers has been set at 18 mg, the amount recommended for nonlactating nonpregnant women. In most cases 18 mg per day should provide sufficient iron to meet a mother's personal needs, once she has replenished prenatal stores by continuing iron supplementation for the first two to three months after her baby is born.

Iodine content of human milk is highly influenced by maternal diet. Nursing mothers should keep iodine levels at the recommended .150 mg by using iodized salt in all foods prepared in the home. Since goiter may occur in persons of any age, the nursing baby must receive adequate iodine intakes to prevent this deficiency disorder. An adequately nourished mother who includes iodized salt in her daily diet will provide her nursing baby with enough iodine to meet or exceed his RDA.

If a mother drinks water that contains at least 1.1 ppm of fluoride, her nursing infant gets enough of this mineral in breast milk to help ensure good dental health. Giving the baby a fluoride supplement seems unwarranted in such cases, especially since excessive fluoride intakes can cause mottling of teeth. In a 1976 publication by the American Academy of Pedodontics Dr. Frederick Parkins, professor of Pedodontics, College of Dentistry, University of Iowa, has written: "Experts question the value of prescribing fluoride supplements to a child younger than six months of age. Research does not show benefits significant enough to justify [risking] the mottling that may occur when young infants receive fluoride supplements." Dr. Stephen Wei, head of Department of Pedodontics at University of Iowa, agrees with Dr. Parkins in view of the fact that most babies below six months of age receive some fluoride in water or baby food. While the totally breast-fed infant under 6 months might possibly benefit from fluoride supplementation, such supplementation is not currently thought necessary. Until transfer of fluoride in breast milk is more completely understood, mothers are advised to rely on Dr. Parkin's opinion.

Reports of zinc concentrations in breast milk vary widely, and the National Research Council has called for reevaluation of zinc content by modern methods. Based on current knowledge of the amount of zinc secreted in each day's milk supply, the RDA for this mineral has been set at 25 mg during lactation.

The winter 1970 cover of *Nutrition Today* featured a photo that brought both praise and condemnation to that journal. The blue-toned photograph depicted a blond-haired young woman nursing a four- to five-month-old baby. Wearing the headband, necklace, and rings of the hippie culture, the stony-eyed mother leaned against a tree trunk, a half-smoked cigarette hanging loosely from her mouth. The cover caption read simply, "Breast Milk." The implications of that cover became obvious when readers turned to the journal's lead article, "Contamination of the Ideal Food." In that article Dr. Jay M. Arena, professor of pediatrics and director of the Poison Control Center at Duke University School of Medicine, explored the many ways in which potentially dangerous elements, including nicotine and marijauna, might enter human milk.

Dr. Arena's overview on the topic should be required reading matter for every doctor and every nursing mother. Earlier generations of breast-feeding women were far less likely to overdose their babies, for they seldom took drugs themselves. In today's pill-for-every-ill society accidental overdosing of nursing infants is an ever-increasing danger. As an avid proponent of breast feeding, Dr. Arena is greatly concerned over indiscriminate use of drugs by lactating women. Most prescription drugs, oral contraceptives, social toxicants, and ecological toxicants cross into the mother's milk. Since toxicity of all drugs is related to the body weight of the recipient, a less-than-lethal dosage for a mother could be fatal to her nursing child.

Clark's rule, a method of relating drug dosage to body weight, can be applied to the nursing pair to determine which fraction of the adult dose of a drug should be safe for an infant. By dividing the child's weight by that of the mother one can determine which fraction of the drug dosage should be safe for the baby. If a 10-pound baby received only 1/12 of the dosage taken by its 120-pound mother, it would receive a full therapeutic dose, the maximum amount that a pediatrician might prescribe for the baby. For example, assuming that the mother took *exactly* the amount of antibiotic that her doctor prescribed and assuming that no more than 1/12 of this particular antibiotic was secreted into the milk, then the baby would receive a therapeutic antibiotic dose—whether or not he needed one. Suppose, however, that the baby *did* need an antibiotic. Most likely his mother would obtain a prescription from her pediatrician. She might or might not think to mention to her baby's doctor the fact that she was also ill and was taking an antibiotic. In such a case the pediatrician's prescription alone might meet the baby's needs; that prescription plus the antibiotic received in mother's milk might mean significant overdosing.

The problem becomes more complex when one realizes that not all drugs pass into the mother's milk in equal proportions. Some are passed on in minute amounts; others in dangerously high amounts. Very little research has been done to determine the extent to which drugs are transferred into a human mother's milk.

Mothers who receive large intramuscular injections of penicillin pass on significant amounts of the drug to their nursing infant. Mothers who take penicillin orally transfer lesser quantities to their breast-fed babies. Radioactive iodine has been shown to cross into breast milk and exert suppressive action on the developing thyroid gland of the nursing infant. Thiouracil administered to a lactating woman could induce goiter in her nursing baby. Bromides, ergot, and anthraguinones are secreted in human milk and may cause problems for the infant in cases of maternal misuse of these drugs.

Though supporting breast-feeding in most cases, Dr. Arena discourages the practice for women who must receive large doses of any drug on a regular basis and for those who are on rare or unusual drugs. Though mothers can safely use many prescription drugs, a lactating woman should be sure that the prescribing physician knows that she is breast feeding. If either doctor or mother questions the safety of a drug, a substitute should be used if possible. In certain cases Dr. Arena's staff at Duke University's Poison Control Center might be able to help make decisions of this kind. In general, Dr. Arena notes: ". . . I am inclined to advise against the use of the following drugs while breast-feeding: any drug or chemical in excessive amounts, diuretics, oral contraceptives, atropine, reserpine, steroids, radioactive preparations, morphine and its derivatives, hallucinogens, anticoagulants, bromides, antithyroid drugs, anthraguinones, dihyrotachysterol and antimetabolites."

New mothers who want to nurse their babies are usually told to avoid oral contraceptives, since the hormones in such preparations inhibit lactation. Some mothers have resumed use of oral contraceptives once lactation has been firmly established, but the practice seems highly questionable in view of the relatively little-known-about effects of oral contraceptives on the nursing infant. Dr. Arena feels that the use of oral contraceptives by a lactating mother could have an unbalancing effect on the developing endocrine system of a nursing baby. Furthermore, mounting evidence as to the potential side effects of the pill makes transmitting such a drug to an infant even more undesirable. It is not likely that a developing child could continue to receive daily jolts of estrogen or progesterone without risk of some imbalance. A government pamphlet warns new mothers that: "After childbirth there is special need to consult your physician before resuming use of the pill. This is especially true if you plan to nurse your baby because the drugs in the pill are known to appear in the milk and the long-range effect on the infant is not known at this time. Furthermore, the pill may cause a decrease in your milk supply."

All current evidence indicates that nursing mothers should avoid use of oral contraceptives.

Labeling alcohol, nicotine, barbituates, marijuana, and other such drugs as social toxicants, Dr. Arena reminds nursing mothers that their babies receive minidoses of all such substances. The alcoholic mother isn't likely to be able to nurse her child, and the mother who drinks only moderately isn't likely to harm the child. Nicotine, one of the most toxic of all drugs, isn't likely to prove deadly to the nursing child of a mother who is a moderate smoker. Dr. Arena's staff advises against heavy smoking while nursing. Barbituates ingested by the mother have not been found harmful to nursing infants. For drugs such as marijuana the verdict is not yet in. Since the most active component of marijuana is fat-soluble, the drug probably passes into breast milk. The long-range effect of minihits of this drug on a nursing baby are not yet known.

While Dr. Arena reported that infants "are in no apparent danger from present levels of DDT in their mother's milk," other pesticides and herbicides currently being used may pose problems for some nursing mothers. In the fall of 1976 mothers in one area of Michigan were urged to give up breast feeding when high levels of PBB (polybrominated biphenyls) were found in their milk. As of October, 1976, the PBB (accidentally added to animal feed in 1974) had been linked to animal deaths and human illness in farm families. Stored in body fat and secreted in breast milk, it reportedly posed grave dangers for newborns.

Nursing women thoughout the country sympathized with the decision faced by the Michigan mothers. It appeared that conscientious mothers in that area had no choice but to give up breast-feeding. Nationwide headlines blared out the warnings against PBB, yet only a few small articles presenting important additional facts were carried by those same newspapers. Ever aware of the potential dangers of ecological toxicants, La Leche League International met with several of the nation's top authorities on toxicants and concluded that there was no real basis for advising against breastfeeding due to PBB contamination. One of those experts, Dr. Mark Thoman, Editor-in-Chief of *AACTION,* official publication of the American Academy of Clinical Toxicology, advised League mothers that the known advantages of breast-feeding "clearly outweigh the theoretical but extremely remote possibility of future problems from minuscule amounts of these substances in mother's milk. It seems obvious that sticking to the known benefits of breastfeeding is the wiser choice."

As of the closing months of 1976, this advice was the latest available through La Leche League. If additional developments cause that opinion to change, LLL will be ready to advise its members and all nursing women of the change. As Marion Tompson, League President, noted, "It's vitally important that any actions taken be neither hasty nor ill-advised."

Mothers who fear that their breast milk may have been contaminted by PBB or any related substance must weigh all available data before deciding whether to cease breastfeeding. A call or letter to La Leche League, Dr. Jay Arena or Dr. Mark Thoman should bring to a concerned mother the latest opinions on this perplexing issue.

Certainly, if there is ever definite evidence that the risks of nursing outweigh its advantages, a mother would be well advised to give up nursing. To insist that "breast is best" when breast milk has been severely contaminated would be to show more interest in the act of breastfeeding than in the health of one's child. The PBB incident and others like it serve as strong reminders that the nursing mother must guard with care the purity of her milk supply

Meeting the Nutrional Need of the Nursing Mother
Translating RDA notations into menus may seem an impossible task for the average nursing mother. Certainly the task would be difficult even for a mother with a degree in chemistry. Fortunately, use of the modified exchange lists presented and explained in Chapter 7 can make menu planning a simple matter for the nursing mother. In fact, nursing mothers who used the exchange system during pregnancy will have no trouble adapting that same system to fit their nutritional needs during lactation. Mothers who did not use this guide during pregnancy should read Chapter 7 before attempting to use the Daily Meal-pattern chart for Lactating Mothers which follows this section.

Once the exchange method of planning is understood, a nursing mother can determine her caloric needs and adapt the Daily Meal Pattern Chart for Lactating Mothers to fit those needs. In adding calories to the basic 2,600-calorie guide she should add *quality* foods, not just empty calories. In subtracting calories she must be sure that all nucleus exchanges given on the "Recommended Minimum Daily Totals" line remain in her diet.

Once she has adapted the Meal Pattern Chart for Lactating to her own caloric needs, the mother can use that chart to determine which foods she should choose from the exchange lists given in chapter 7. She can then combine those foods into appetizing menus and snacks, following the instructions given in that chapter.

To make meal planning easier during those first busy weeks of baby's life, a full week's menus and snacks for the lactating woman can be obtained by adding specific protein foods to the 7 prenatal menu plans in Part III. Since converting recipes to the exchange system can be a time-consuming procedure, each day's menus and snacks feature recipes that are included in the recipe section in Part III. Later a nursing mother can convert her own favorite recipes to the exchange system, following the instructions given in Chapter 7. She should have no trouble meeting RDA standards.

The menus and snacks in Part III should serve as a reminder that a nursing mother should be able to enjoy many different foods—from spicy barbeques to oriental dishes. Only if repeated experiments seem to indicate that a certain food or certain food combinations cause discomfort for her baby need a mother consider giving up those foods while nursing. She should also remember that what seemed to cause colic for a four-week-old baby may not bother the same baby at six months of age.

During weaning months, caloric intakes for the nursing mother should be readjusted, as explained earlier, to reflect diminished milk production.

Since post-lactation needs are similar to the postpartum needs of the non-nursing mother, the nursing mother can consult chapter II after she has weaned her baby.

DAILY MEAL PATTERN FOR 2600 CALORIE LACTATION DIET

	MILK			Milk Kcal Per Meal Or Snack	VEGETABLE			Vegetable Kcal Per Meal Or Snack	FRUIT		Fruit Kcal Per Meal Or Snack	BREAD		Bread Kcal Per Meal Or Snack	MEAT			Meat Kcal Per Meal Or Snack	FAT	Fat Kcal Per Meal Or Snack	Total Kcal Per Snack
	A 80	B 125	C 170		A 25	B 25	C 25		A 40	B 40		A 70	B 70		A 55	B 77	C 100		45		
Breakfast	1½			188					1		40	2		140	1	1		177	2	90	635
Mid-morning Snack	½			63								1		70	1			77			210
Lunch	1			125	1	1		50	1		40	2		140	3			231	2	90	676
Afternoon Snack	½			63																	
Dinner	1½			188	1		1	50	2		80	3	1	280	4			308	2	90	996
Evening Snack									1		40	`									
Actual Daily Totals Per Exchange	5			627	2	1	1	100	3	2	200	8	1	630	9	1		793	6	270	2620
Recommended Minimum Daily Totals	5			varies 400-850	2		1	75	1		40	3	1	280	8-9			varies 495-900	as needed to meet calorie requirements		Maximum 2600 Calories

UNDERSTANDING AND MEETING THE NUTRITIONAL NEEDS OF THE NONNURSING MOTHER

[After the birth of her baby] several goals may be accomplished -- nutritional depletions of pregnancy and/or lactation may be rehabilitated, weight may be brought to desired levels, and nutritional health of the entire family may be promoted.

(Nutrition in Maternal Health Care,
Committee on Nutrition, American College
of Obstetricians and Gynecologists,
Chicago, Illinois, 1974)

Though the nursing mother's needs have been discussed in greater detail within this guide, the needs of the nonnursing mother are just as important. Though her body will no longer be physically supporting a new life, her emotional, mental, and physical reserves will be taxed in other ways by the responsibilities of motherhood. She should begin to replenish nutritional depletions, bring her weight to the desired level, and promote the nutritional health of her family. The following discussion offers guidance in meeting all three of these goals.

Replenishing Nutritional Depletions
The American College of Obstetricians and Gynecologists has advised its members to suggest that new mothers continue iron supplements at the prenatal rate for two to three months. Iron stores are quite likely to be low after pregnancy, even if a woman has been taking a prenatal iron supplement. Replenishing those stores means that a woman is less likely to be iron-deficient during the months to come as the returning menstrual periods once more take iron from her body.

Women who use oral contraceptives may have a greater risk of certain vitamin deficiencies than do other women. According to the American College of Obstetricians and Gynecologists biochemical evidence suggest increased needs for Vitamins B_2, B_6, B_{12}, C and B_9 (folic acid) as well as certain trace minerals. Since an otherwise healthy woman is unlikely to be under close medical supervision when not pregnant during her reproductive years, she must become her own caretaker. By making sure that her diet contains recommended daily allowances of the above vitamins she lessens her chances of deficiency, even if use of the pill increases those chances. If any deficiency symptoms do occur, she should report them to her doctor and ask his advice on the matter.

Women who use intrauterine contraceptive devices (IUCDs) often experience an increase in menstrual blood loss. Since two-thirds of menstruating women are unable to accumulate adequate stores of iron, the IUCD user should pay special attention to iron-rich foods. If iron-deficiency-anemia symptoms appear, she should seek her doctor's advice. In some cases iron supplements may need to be prescribed.

If a woman has followed a sound prenatal diet, she should not be deficient in major vitamins and minerals, and continuing a nutritionally sound eating program is the best way to make sure that deficiencies do not develop. By following a modified version of her prenatal diet a new mother can adjust calorie intakes to fit her postpartum needs yet maintain nutritionally sound eating habits.

Bringing Weight to Desired Levels
If a young woman began pregnancy at ideal weight for height and gained no more than the recommended number of pounds, she can probably deduct 300 calories from her prenatal diet (the number that she added to meet the caloric demands of pregnancy) and with exercise enjoy a gradual but steady return to prepregnancy weight.

If she began pregnancy at lower than average weight for height, she may choose to retain the 300 extra calories to help add the desired number of pounds. With her doctor's supervision she can set a weight-gain goal and continue prenatal caloric intakes until she reaches the chosen weight. Thereafter, by gradually decreasing calories she can find her maintenance level, the calorie level at which she can keep a fairly constant weight.

The woman who was obese before pregnancy began and/or gained excessive amounts during pregnancy should consider beginning a weight-loss regimen around two to four weeks after delivery. With her doctor's help she can adjust caloric intakes downward to a level at which she should lose approximately one pound per week. She can omit the necessary fat and bread exchanges, leaving in her diet the variety of vegetables, fruits, meats, and milk products necessary to ensure adequate intakes of vitamins, minerals, proteins, and carbohydrates.

To lose one pound per week, approximately 500 calories should be omitted from one's daily intake at maintenance level. The exchange diet allows a nonpregnant woman to make this large a reduction in calories without danger of losing vital nutrients. Of course, for a postpartum woman, this means a rather sudden reduction of 800 calories per day (300 deducted after baby's birth, 500 more at whatever time the doctor agrees to the start of a weight-loss regimen). To make this large a reduction does take will power, and dropping 300, then 100 more calories per day up to a total of 800 is probably easier than dropping all 800 at once. The Daily Meal Pattern Chart for Postpartum Diet on the following page, gives one pattern for a 1,600-calorie diet that maintains all vital nutrients yet allows for a loss of approximately one pound per week of body fat. Since such a diet does not mean starving oneself, most women should be able to adjust their intakes to fit the maximums indicated on the chart.

As mentioned earlier, if one goes below the 1,800-calorie level, it is extremely difficult to maintain nutritional balance without drastic reductions in sugar, alcohol, and fat intakes. In planning a diet of 1,600 calories, for example, one must be very careful to omit almost all empty, high-calorie foods. Such foods provide little more than calories, and they should *not* be allowed to replace more nutritious foods.

Below 1,600 calories maintaining nutritional balance is so difficult that a woman should try such a diet only under close medical supervision. Women who fail to lose weight at 1,600 calories should try exercise as a means of lowering intake beyond this level. Proper exercise can reduce the daily calorie loads to levels low enough to cause weight loss at the desired rate. Postpartum exercises can help to tone muscles and consume some calories, but more strenuous exercises may be needed to effect significant weight losses. Before beginning very strenuous exercises a woman should check with her doctor to be sure that no physical limitations make such exercises unwise in her particular case.

Before beginning any weight-reduction program a woman should seek her doctor's advice as to the amount, rate, and method of weight loss that he feels best suits her particular needs. Her doctor might chose to refer her to a diet counselor or nutritionist.

Promoting Nutritional Health of the Entire Family

The exchange plans presented for prenatal, lactation, and postpartum diets can be modified to meet the needs of the entire family. By consulting the complete Recommended Daily Dietary Allowances Chart published by The National Research Council, a woman can learn the calorie, protein, vitamin, and mineral needs of each member of her family. In most cases her experience in using the exchange system will enable her to translate RDA notations into exchanges and to devise an exchange meal-pattern chart for each family member.

By continuing to use the knowledge that she has gained while following the prenatal, lactation, and postpartum guidelines within this book a mother will be granting her children a priceless legacy: sound eating habits that will form the basis for a lifetime of good health.

DAILY MEAL PATTERN CHART FOR 1600 CALORIE POSTPARTUM DIET

	MILK				VEGETABLE				FRUIT			BREAD			MEAT				FAT		Total Kcal Per Meal Or
	A 80	B 125	C 170	Milk Kcal Per Meal Or Snack	A 25	B 25	C 25	Vegetable Kcal Per Meal Or Snack	A 40	B 40	Fruit Kcal Per Meal Or Snack	A 70	B 70	Bread Kcal Per Meal Or Snack	A 55	B 77	C 100	Meat Kcal Per Meal Or Snack	45	Fat Kcal Per Meal Or Snack	Snack
Breakfast	1			80					1		40	1		70	1	1		177	1	45	412
Mid-morning Snack																					
Lunch	1			80	1	1		50	1		40	1		70	2			154	2	90	484
Afternoon Snack																					
Dinner	1			80	1		1	50	2		80	2	1	210	4			308	2	90	818
Evening Snack																					
Actual Daily Totals Per Exchange			3	240	2	1	1	100	3	1	160	4	1	350	7			539	5	225	1614
Recommended Minimum Daily Totals			3	240-510	2			75	1		40				7-8			330-800	as needed to meet calorie requirements		Maximum 1600 Calories

Part III

MENUS AND RECIPES

FOR

PRENATAL AND

POSTPARTUM DIETS

Therapeutic diets and nutritional counseling, whether
directed toward correcting a physiologic deviation arising
in pregnancy or toward improving long-term food habits,
involve the difficult task of changing long-entrenched
eating patterns. [For optimum results one should]
obtain baseline information for evaluating later
deviations . . .

Jean Mayer, Johanna T. Dwyer,
Howard N. Jacobson, and Bobbie K. Hutchins
(*Post-Graduate Medicine*, October 1970)

MENUS

The seven menus given in this section meet RDA Standards for a prenatal diet of 2,400 calories. By adding the snacks marked by a double asterisk (**), these menus can be adjusted to meet RDA standards for a 2,600 calorie lactation diet. Entrees whose recipes appear in this book are marked by a single asterisk.

DAY 1
MENUS AND SNACKS FOR 2400 CALORIE PRENATAL DIET

BREAKFAST:
    8 oz. 2% Milk   2 Whole Wheat/Fruit Pancakes*
    4 oz. Orange Juice   1 cup Coffee or Tea, if desired

MID-MORNING SNACK:
    4 oz. Tomato Juice
    1½ oz. Smoked Swiss Cheese

LUNCH:
    Stonehouse Soup*
    Finnish Farmer's Whole Wheat Bread* (⅛ of 10" circle) with margarine
    8 oz. 2% Milk
    1 Fresh Peach or Nectarine

AFTERNOON SNACK:
    1 8 oz. carton low-fat, fruit-flavored Yogurt**

DINNER:
    Barbara's Beef Curry*
    Saffron Rice and Peas*
    Green Apple Green Salad with Orange Dressing*
    Tea or Coffee
    Fruit Flambeau Finale*

EVENING SNACK:
—

DAY 2
MENUS AND SNACKS FOR 2400 CALORIE PRENATAL DIET

BREAKFAST:
    8 oz. 2% Milk
    1 Oatmeal-Nut Waffle* with honey, butter and applesauce
    2 oz. Canadian Bacon
    Coffee or Tea (if desired)

MID-MORNING SNACK:
    2 Plums (⅛ if applesauce was used on waffle)
    2 oz. Cheddar Cheese**

*Recipe appears in recipe section   **Add for 2600 calorie lactation diet only

LUNCH:
    Vegetable Yogurt Salad*
    1 Sesame Seed Snack*
    Iced Tea

AFTERNOON SNACK:
    Nectarine Shake*

DINNER:
    3-Meat Bar-B-Que*   French Bread
    Swart's Baked Beans*   Iced Tea
    Lettuce Salad   Watermelon (2 cups)

EVENING SNACK:
    8 oz. Hot Cocoa

DAY 3
MENUS AND SNACKS FOR 2400 CALORIE PRENATAL DIET

BREAKFAST:
    4 oz. Orange Juice
    Breakfast Fruit Parfait*
    Coffee or Tea
    8 oz. 2% Milk**

MID-MORNING SNACK:
    4 oz. Vegetable Juice Cocktail
    ½ oz. Farmer's Cheese**

LUNCH:
    Colombo Fish Stew*
    Finnish Farmer's Whole Wheat Bread* (⅛ of 10" round)
    8 oz. 2% Milk *or*
    1 oz. Cheddar or Swiss Cheese

AFTERNOON SNACK:
    —

DINNER:
    Cheese Soup*
    Cornish Hens with Fruited Rice Stuffing*
    Asparagus with Sour Cream Sauce*
    Tomato-Ripe Olive Salad*
    Tea or Coffee
    Orange-Date Bread*

EVENING SNACK:
    6 oz. Hot Cocoa

*Recipe appears in recipe section   **Add for 2600 calorie lactation diet only

DAY 4
MENUS AND SNACKS FOR 2400 CALORIE PRENATAL DIET

BREAKFAST:
 8 oz. % Milk
 1 slice Canteloupe (¼ small)
 Texas Ham Omelette*
 1 slice Whole Wheat Toast with jam and butter
 Coffee or Tea, if desired

MID-MORNING SNACK:
 8 oz. plain low-fat Yogurt**
 4 oz. Applesauce**

LUNCH:
 Avocado Open-face Sandwich*
 8 oz. Vegetable Juice Cocktail

AFTERNOON SNACK:
 Banana Malt*

DINNER:
 Donna's Sweet and Sour Pork*
 Lettuce and Chinese Vegetable Salad* with Soy dressing
 Coffee or Tea
 Zucchini Bread*

DAY 5
MENUS AND SNACKS FOR 2400 CALORIE PRENATAL DIET

BREAKFAST:
 4 oz. Orange Juice
 8 oz. 2% Milk
 Whole Wheat Muffins* with ½ cup Applesauce
 2 small Sausage Links
 Coffee or Tea, if desired

MID-MORNING SNACK:
 ½ cup Cottage Cheese**   1 Peach**

LUNCH:
 Tarragon Tuna Salad*   8 oz. 2% Milk
 Rye Crisps (3)   2 Molasses Cookies*

DINNER:
 Bar-B-Qued Chicken Quarters   Tea or Coffee
 3-Lettuce Salad   1 cup Ice Milk with Strawberries
 Lombardy Green Tart*

*Recipe appears in recipe section   **Add for 2600 calorie lactation diet only

DAY 6
MENUS AND SNACKS FOR 2400 CALORIE PRENATAL DIET

BREAKFAST:
Strawberry Shake*

MID-MORNING SNACK:
8 oz. plain low-fat Yogurt
1 Orange**

LUNCH:
Salmon Salad*   Carrot Sticks   8 oz. 2% Milk

DINNER:
Chicken Della Robbia*   Chalah Bread (1 slice)*
Fluffy White Rice (½ cup)   Cranberry Bread (2 slices)*
Green Beans with Water Chestnuts   Coffee or Tea

EVENING SNACK:
8 oz. hot Cocoa**

DAY 7
MENUS AND SNACKS FOR 2400 CALORIE PRENATAL DIET

BREAKFAST:
Fortified Peanut Butter-Orange Bread* (1 slice)
8 oz. 2% Milk
Coffee or Tea, if desired

MID-MORNING SNACK:
Whole Wheat Peanut Butter Sandwich**
8 oz. 2% Milk**

LUNCH:
Fried Rice*
Lettuce-Chinese Vegetable Salad*
8 oz. 2% Milk

AFTERNOON SNACK:
4 oz. Vegetable Juice Cocktail

DINNER:
Gingered Beef and Vegetables*   Coffee or Tea
New Potatoes*   1 cup Ice Milk**
Tropical Salad*

*Recipe appears in recipe section
**Add full amount for 2600 calorie lactation diet only. For 2400 calorie prenatal diet, include only
  ½ sandwich, 4 oz. milk, and ½ cup ice milk.

RECIPES

Since the following recipes are keyed for use in exchange-type meal plans, they are arranged in six exchange sections—milk, vegetable, fruit, meat, bread and fat. The group in which a recipe appears depends upon its exchange value. For example, Texas Ham Omelette for Two (3 meat, ½ milk, 1 fat, ¼ vegetable A/C) appears under meat exchanges, while New Potatoes (2 bread, 1½ fat) appears under bread exchanges. The comprehensive index also allows one to find recipes according to their exact titles and/or chief ingredients.

Many of the dishes given in the following pages were devised by homemakers who seldom use cook books or write down recipes, homemakers who cook by the "dash of this" and "pinch of that" method. Though they were willing to translate their recipes into measurements in order to share them, they stressed freedom to experiment as a key to their years of cooking success.

The recipes are introduced, then, as a starting point for the woman who wants to try dishes which go a long way toward helping meet her family's nutritional needs. They carry with them the invitation to experiment—in short, the invitation to turn the words and numbers of the printed page into delicious dishes tailored to fit the likes and needs of a particular family.

MILK EXCHANGES

Banana Malt
Servings: 1
Exchanges per serving: 1½ milk, ½ fat, 2 fruit A

Ingredients:
8 ounces 2% milk
1 ripe banana, quartered
1 tablespoon malted-milk powder
4 ounces (½ cup) vanilla ice milk

Directions:
1. Place milk, banana, malted-milk powder, and ice milk in blender container.
2. Blend at high speed for 10 to 12 seconds.

Nectarine Shake
Servings: 1
Exchanges per serving: 1 milk, 1 fruit

Ingredients:
1 nectarine, peeled and halved
8 ounces 2% milk
1 teaspoon honey
Dash of nutmeg

Directions:
1. Place nectarine, milk, honey, and nutmeg in blender.
2. Mix to desired consistency.

Strawberry Shake
Servings: 1
Exchanges per serving: 1 milk, 1 meat, 1 fruit C, ½ bread

Ingredients:
8 ounces 2% milk
1 egg
10 strawberries
2 teaspoons honey
¼ teaspoon vanilla flavoring

Directions:
1. Place ingredients in blender container.
2. Blend until smooth and serve immediately.

Cheese Soup
Servings: 4
Exchanges per serving: ¾ fat, 1½ milk

Ingredients:
2 tablespoons chopped onion
1 tablespoon butter
1 tablespoon flour
2 bouillon cubes
¾ cup water
2 cups 2% milk
1 cup grated cheddar cheese
Salt and paprika to taste

Directions:
1. Sauté chopped onions in melted butter until transparent.
2. Dissolve 2 bouillon cubes in ¾ cup boiling water.
3. Stir flour into onion/butter mixture and add broth mixture, blending well.
4. Bring sauce mixture to a boil, then add 2 cups of milk. Heat but do not boil.
5. Slowly add 1 cup grated cheese and stir until melted. Add salt and paprika to taste.

Vegetable-yogurt Salad
Servings: 1
Exchanges per serving: 1 milk B, 1 vegetable C, 1½ vegetable B

Ingredients:
1 8-ounce carton plain, low-fat yogurt
1 medium tomato, chopped
1 small cucumber, chopped
1 small red onion, chopped
Dash of cinnamon
Salt and pepper to taste

Directions:
1. Chop all vegetables and sprinkle with cinnamon, salt, and pepper.
2. Mix vegetables and yogurt.

Avocado Open-face Sandwich
Servings: 1
Exchanges per serving: 1 bread, 1 vegetable B, ½ vegetable A, ½ vegetable C, 1 milk, 2 fat

Ingredients:
1 slice whole-wheat bread
1 teaspoon margarine
¼ cup shredded carrots
¼ cup sliced scallions
⅛ cup sliced mushrooms
½ small tomato, sliced
⅛ cup bean sprouts
1 ounce Swiss or Monterey Jack cheese, sliced
⅛ ounce 4" avocado, sliced

Directions:
1. Butter bread.
2. Stack next 6 ingredients onto bread, ending with slices of cheese.
3. Top with avocado slices.

Breakfast Parfait
Servings: 2
Exchanges per serving: ¾ milk B, 1¼ fruit A, 1 bread, ¼ fruit B, 1 fat

Ingredients:
½ cup low-fat plain yogurt
½ cup small-curd cottage cheese
½ cup applesauce
¼ cup fresh orange segments
¼ cup toasted wheat germ
½ small apple, unpeeled and chopped
½ medium banana, sliced

Directions:
1. Mix yogurt, cottage cheese, and applesauce.
2. Alternate layers of yogurt mixture with layers of orange, wheat germ, apple, and banana.
3. Top each parfait with 1 tablespoon chopped nuts.

VEGETABLE EXCHANGES

Asparagus with Sour-cream Sauce
Servings: 4
Exchanges per serving: 1 fat, 1 vegetable A

Ingredients:
2 bunches fresh asparagus or 2 10-ounce packages frozen asparagus
½ cup sour cream
4 teaspoons vinegar
1 tablespoon sugar
Pinch of salt

Directions:
1. Steam asparagus and drain. Arrange in bottom of 1½-quart casserole.
2. Mix sour cream, vinegar, sugar, and salt. Pour mixture over hot asparagus.

Green Beans with Water Chestnuts
Servings: 7 to 8 ½-cup servings
Exchanges per serving: 1-1/3 vegetable B, ¾ fat

Ingredients:
2 9-ounce packages frozen French-style green beans
1 8½-ounce can water chestnuts
⅛ cup butter (2 tablespoons)
½ teaspoon salt
¼ teaspoon pepper
½ teaspoon marjoram leaves
½ teaspoon tarragon leaves
2 teaspoons lemon juice

Directions:
1. Cook beans following package directions.
2. Drain water chestnuts and cut into very thin slices.
3. Melt butter in a skillet and stir in spices and lemon juice.
4. Add water chestnuts and seasoned butter to beans.
5. Toss to mix well, heat to steaming, and serve immediately.

Lombardy Green Tart
Servings: 4
Exchanges per serving: 1 bread, 2 fat, 1 milk, 1½ vegetable B, 1 vegetable A

Ingredients:
1 deep-dish 10" pie shell, baked at 425° for 10 minutes and allowed to cool.
2 cups cottage cheese (small-curd)
1 medium zucchini, cut in ¼" pieces
2 stalks celery, cut in ⅛" pieces
1 bunch scallions, chopped (green part only)
1 box frozen, chopped spinach, cooked, thoroughly drained, and squeezed dry
2 tablespoons fresh, minced parsley (or 1 tablespoon parsley flakes)
¾ teaspoon marjoram

¾ teaspoon thyme
4 eggs, slightly beaten
¼ teaspoon salt
Pepper to taste

Directions:
1. Combine all ingredients in a deep bowl.
2. Pour into baked pie shell and bake at 375° for 30 to 40 minutes.
3. Serve hot or cold.

Carrot-raisin Salad
Servings: 6
Exchanges per serving: 1 vegetable B, ½ fruit

Ingredients:
6 carrots
1½ cups raisins
¼ cup orange juice
2 teaspoons mayonnaise
½ teaspoon salt

Directions:
1. Grate carrots and mix well with raisins.
2. Mix orange juice, mayonnaise, and salt.
3. Add dressing to carrot mixture and serve.

Chef's Salad
Servings: 4
Exchanges per serving: ½ vegetable C, 1 vegetable A, 1 vegetable B, 1 meat, 1 fat

Ingredients:
½ head iceberg lettuce
1 bunch endive or escarole
2 carrots, thinly sliced with vegetable peeler
1 red onion, sliced and separated into rings
2 medium tomatoes, cut into wedges
8 unpeeled, sliced radishes
2 sliced hard-cooked eggs
½ cup grated cheddar cheese
Freshly ground black pepper to taste
½ teaspoon basil

Directions:
1. Toss shredded lettuce, endive or escarole, sliced carrots, red onion rings, tomato wedges, and sliced radishes in a large salad bowl. Add favorite vinegar-and-oil dressing and toss again lightly.
2. Arrange hard-cooked eggs on top of salad mixture and sprinkle with grated cheese.
3. Grind black pepper over cheese and sprinkle salad lightly with basil.

Tomato-ripe-olive Salad
Servings: 4
Exchanges per serving: 1 vegetable C, ½ fat

Ingredients:
4 medium tomatoes, cut in wedges
12 ripe olives
Basil, salt, and fresh ground pepper to taste

Directions:
1. Arrange tomato wedges from one tomato and three ripe olives on each salad plate.
2. Add salt, pepper, and basil to taste.

Lettuce-and-Chinese-vegetable Salad
Servings: 8
Exchanges per serving: ¼ vegetable B, ¾ bread, ¾ vegetable A

Ingredients:
½ cup bean sprouts
10 medium mushrooms, sliced
¾ cup sliced celery
1 bunch spinach (1 cup, torn)
1 bunch leaf lettuce (2 cups, torn)
¼ cup water
½ cup sugar
½ cup vinegar
½ teaspoon celery seed
½ teaspoon mustard seed
Dash soy sauce

Directions:
1. Clean sprouts and blanch in boiling, salted water for 2 to 3 minutes. Drain and cool.
2. Gently toss sprouts, mushrooms, celery, spinach, and lettuce.
3. Mix water, sugar, vinegar, celery seed, mustard seed, and soy sauce.
4. Drizzle dressing over salad just before serving. Toss lightly.

FRUIT EXCHANGE

Green-apple Green Salad
Servings: 4 to 6
Exchanges per serving: 1 fruit A, 1 vegetable A, ½ fat

Ingredients:
½ head iceberg lettuce, shredded
1 bunch red-leaf lettuce, shredded
2 tart green apples, chopped
½ cup raisins
¼ cup orange juice
1 teaspoon brown sugar
1 teaspoon lemon juice
1 teaspoon mayonnaise

Directions:
1. Prepare dressing by mixing orange juice, brown sugar, lemon juice, and mayonnaise.
2. Toss lettuce, green apples, and raisins in a large salad bowl.
3. Drizzle with orange dressing and toss again.

Tropical Salad
Servings: 6
Exchanges per serving: ½ fruit C, 1 fruit A, 2-1/3 fat

Ingredients:
1 avocado
1 papaya
1 mango
2 tablespoons vegetable oil
3 tablespoons lemon juice
1 tablespoon water
½ teaspoon lime juice
¼ teaspoon salt
⅛ teaspoon pepper
⅛ teaspoon ginger
1 cup seedless green grapes
1 banana, sliced

Directions:
1. Place peeled, sliced avocado, papaya, and mango in shallow dish.
2. Mix oil, water, juice, salt, pepper, and ginger in shaker or jar and shake well to blend.
3. Pour dressing over fruit, cover, and refrigerate for 1 to 3 hours.
4. Drain dressing from fruit. Spoon fruit into individual serving dishes and top with grapes and banana slices.

Fruit Flambeau Finale
Servings: 8
Exchanges per serving: 1½ fruit

Ingredients:
½ cantaloupe cut in 1" wedges
4 peaches, peeled and quartered
2 bananas, cut in rounds
24 Thompson seedless grapes
2 oranges, peeled and sectioned
2/3 cup Bacardi 151-proof rum
1/3 cup Triple Sec (or Orange Curaçao, Blue Curaçao, or other orange liqueur)
5 to 10 fresh mint sprigs

Directions:
1. Prepare fruit as described above. Place fruit in covered lazy-susan containers and refrigerate during dinner hour.
2. Warm rum and liqueur mixture and pour into stainless-steel, silver, or heat-proof earthenware container.
3. Arrange cold fruit dishes around lazy-susan center and garnish each fruit dish with one or two sprigs of mint. Place rum mixture in center of lazy-susan and ignite.
4. Each person uses a fondue fork to spear fruit and cook in flaming liqueur. Calories flame away, leaving the flavor of the rum-liqueur mixture.

MEAT EXCHANGE

Texas Ham Omelet
Servings: 2
Exchanges per serving: 3 meat, 1 fat, ¼ vegetable A/C, ½ milk

Ingredients:
½ cup cubed ham (2 ounces)
4 eggs
¼ cup milk
¼ cup grated cheddar cheese
1 tablespoon chopped green chili peppers
1 tablespoon chopped scallions
1 tablespoon chopped tomato
Salt and pepper to taste

Directions:
1. Place eggs and milk into large bowl and mix thoroughly with fork.
2. Add chili peppers, scallions, and tomatoes and mix well. Add salt and pepper to taste. Stir again.
3. Heat griddle or large frying pan. Rub end of margarine stick over griddle lightly.
4. Slowly pour omelet mixture onto griddle. When eggs begin to puff and dry around edges, halve omelet and turn halves carefully.
5. Remove to plate and garnish with fresh tomato wedges and parsley sprigs if desired.

Colombo Fish Stew
Servings: 4
Exchanges per serving: 4 meat, 1 bread B, 1¼ vegetable B

Ingredients:
1 pound fresh or frozen fish, cut into 2" cubes
4 small potatoes, cut into 2" cubes
3 large carrots, cut into 2" lengths
2 small onions, quartered
¼ teaspoon salt
2 to 3 cups water
Pepper to taste
1 teaspoon margarine
1 tablespoon chopped onion
1 tablespoon chopped celery
3 whole cloves
3 whole cardamom
1 tablespoon flour
1 teaspoon vinegar

Directions:
1. Place water and salt in saucepan and bring to rolling boil. Drop in fish cubes and boil until tender. Drain fish cubes and set aside. Save water.
2. Cut vegetables into appropriate sizes. Boil in fish water until tender.
3. Melt margarine in heavy skillet and sauté chopped onions and celery until tender. Add cardamom and cloves and sauté for 3 or 4 minutes.
4. Dissolve flour in ½ cup of the water in which fish and vegetables were boiled. Add flour mixture to onions and celery and blend well. Add drained fish and vegetables and mix lightly.
5. Add pepper to taste and additional salt if needed. Simmer for a few minutes or until stew reaches desired consistency.
6. Add vinegar, mix lightly, and serve.

Stonehouse Soup
Servings: 8
Exchanges per serving: 4 meat, 1/3 vegetable B, 2/3 bread

Ingredients:
1 2-pound fryer, cut up, or 2 pounds chicken (bony pieces, backs, necks, wings)
8 cups water
1 carrot, sliced
1 stalk celery with leaves
1 onion, pierced with 6 to 8 whole cloves
1 bay leaf
6 whole black peppercorns
1 teaspoon salt
1 pound pork sausage
1 can vegetable soup
1 can red kidney beans, washed and dried
2 cups shredded cabbage
½ cup uncooked rice

Directions:
1. Place chicken pieces in Dutch oven and add water, carrot, celery, onion with cloves, bay leaf, peppercorns, and salt. Bring to a boil, cover, and simmer 2 hours.
2. Remove bones from chicken and return meat to Dutch oven. Strain broth and put strained broth over meat in Dutch oven.
3. Brown sausage thoroughly in skillet and pour off excess fat.
4. Add sausage, soup, and drained beans to Dutch oven and bring to a boil.
5. Add cabbage and rice, return to boiling point, and simmer until rice is tender (about 20 minutes).

Salmon Salad
Servings: 4
Exchanges per serving: 1 milk, 3¾ meat, 1 bread, 1 vegetable C, 1½ vegetable B, ¾ vegetable A, 1 fat

Ingredients:
1 can salmon (15½ ounces)
2 medium potatoes, cubed, boiled, and drained
1 head cauliflower or 1 package frozen cauliflower, cooked and drained
1 10-ounce package frozen artichoke hearts, cooked and drained
½ cup chopped scallions
1 cup chopped celery
1 tablespoon olive oil
1 tablespoon lemon juice
Salt and pepper to taste
½ teaspoon oregano
4 ounces (1 cup grated) cheddar cheese
4 large lettuce leaves

Directions:
1. Clean, debone, and skin salmon. Place salmon in bottom of bowl and crumble.
2. Add chopped green onions and celery and toss slightly.
3. Pour hot, drained vegetables onto salmon mixture, tossing lightly once more.
4. Add olive oil, lemon juice, salt, pepper, and oregano and toss again.
5. Add cheese and toss once more.
6. Spoon salmon salad onto lettuce leaves on individual salad plates.

Tarragon Tuna Salad
Servings: 2 to 3
Exchanges per serving: 3 medium meat, ½ vegetable A, 1 vegetable C, 2 fat

Ingredients:
1 9¼-ounce can tuna
½ cup diced celery
⅛ cup sweet-pickle relish

¼ teaspoon pepper
¼ teaspoon dry mustard
⅛ teaspoon tarragon leaves
3 scallions, chopped
2 teaspoons lemon juice
¼ cup mayonnaise
2 hard-cooked eggs, sliced
2 small tomatoes, cut in wedges
3 large lettuce leaves

Directions:
1. Drain and flake tuna.
2. Add celery and relish.
3. Combine remaining ingredients in a separate bowl, mixing well. Add to tuna, mixing well.
4. Serve on crisp lettuce leaves. Garnish with eggs and tomato wedges. This salad may also be used as a sandwich filling.

Three-meat Barbecue
Servings: 8
Exchanges per serving: 5 meat

Ingredients:
4 leg-thigh chicken pieces or 4 legs and 4 thighs
4 pork steaks, halved
2 pounds beef spareribs
1 18-ounce jar Kraft hickory-smoked barbecue sauce

Directions:
A. Outdoor-cooking method:
  1. Marinate meat in barbecue sauce for 3 or more hours.
  2. Grill for 25 to 35 minutes over hot coals, turning and basting at least twice with barbecue sauce. Close grill hood during cooking time or use hood fashioned from aluminum foil and wire. Keep cooked pieces in warm oven if limited grill space prevents cooking all at once.
B. Oven-cooked method:
  1. Wrap pork, chicken, and beef ribs in separate foil packages. Pour generous amounts of barbecue sauce over contents of each package and seal foil tightly.
  2. Bake at 350° for 1 hour.

Fried Rice
Servings: 3 to 4
Exchanges per serving: 1¼ meat, ¾ fat, 1 vegetable B, 1 bread

Ingredients:
½ cup diced ham, chicken, pork, or beef (cooked)
1 tablespoon margarine

1 4½-ounce can mushroom stems and pieces
2 tablespoons chopped scallions
2 cups cold cooked rice
2 to 3 tablespoons soy sauce
1 egg, well beaten

Directions:
1. Fry meat lightly in margarine.
2. Add mushrooms, scallions, cold rice, and soy sauce.
3. Cook over low heat for 10 minutes.
4. Add well-beaten egg and cook for 5 minutes longer, stirring frequently.
5. Serve immediately.

Donna's Sweet-and-sour Pork
Servings: 8
Exchanges per serving: 6 meat, 2 bread, 1 fruit A, 1 vegetable B

Ingredients:
3¾ pounds pork steak (1" cubes)
¾ cup flour
1 tablespoon plus 1 teaspoon ginger
½ cup salad oil
2 cans (13½ ounces total) pineapple chunks, drained, reserving syrup
½ cup vinegar
½ cup soy sauce
1 tablespoon Worcestershire sauce
¾ cups sugar
1 tablespoon salt
¾ teaspoon pepper
2 small green peppers, cut into strips
1 can (1 pound) bean sprouts, drained
2 cans (5 ounces each) water chestnuts, drained and thinly sliced
2 tablespoons chili sauce

Directions:
1. Trim excess fat from pork. Combine half the flour and ginger in paper bag. Place 3 pieces of pork at a time in bag. Shake well to coat pieces.
2. Heat oil in large, heavy skillet or Dutch oven. Brown pork on all sides and remove pieces as they brown.
3. Add water to pineapple syrup to measure 1¾ cup liquid and gradually stir remaining flour into water.
4. Stir flour mixture, vinegar, soy sauce, and Worcestershire sauce into pork drippings. Heat to boiling, stirring constantly. Boil 1 minute.
5. Stir in sugar, salt, pepper, and meat. Cover and simmer 1 hour or until meat is tender, stirring occasionally.
6. Add pineapple and green pepper and cook uncovered 10 minutes.
7. Stir in bean sprouts, water chestnuts, and chili sauce and cook 5 minutes longer.
8. Serve over rice (½ cup rice = 1 bread exchange).

Barbara's Beef Curry
Servings: 4
Exchanges per serving: 6 meat, ½ fat, ½ vegetable **B**

Ingredients:
2 tablespoons shortening
1 large onion, finely chopped
1 clove garlic, minced
2 pounds boneless top-round steak, cubed
2 large onions, finely chopped
1 tablespoon ground coriander
½ teaspoon ground pepper
½ teaspoon ground turmeric
½ teaspoon ground red chili
½ teaspoon ground cumin seed
⅛ teaspoon ground ginger
1 cup water
½ cup thick coconut milk or 1 tablespoon flour dissolved in ½ cup water

Directions:
1. Melt shortening in large skillet and sauté 1 chopped onion and minced garlic clove until onion is transparent.
2. Mix cubed beef with remaining onion, coriander, pepper, turmeric, chili, cumin, and ginger.
3. Add meat mixture to sautéed onions and cook over medium heat for 4 to 5 minutes.
4. Add 1 cup water. Simmer gently, with pan covered, until meat is tender.
5. 10 minutes before serving add salt to taste and thicken with coconut milk or flour mixture.

Gingered Beef and Vegetables
Servings: 4
Exchanges per serving: ½ bread, 1½ fat, 4½ meat, 1 vegetable **A**

Ingredients:
1½ pounds boneless sirloin steak
½ cup soy sauce
2 tablespoons honey
½ cup red wine
Dash garlic powder
Small knob of fresh ginger, grated (about 1 tablespoon)
Water to cover beef
2 tablespoons vegetable oil
1 bunch (2 cups shredded) spinach

Directions:
1. Partially freeze steak, then slice in small strips about 2" long.
2. Mix soy sauce, honey, wine, garlic, ginger, and enough water to cover the beef. Pour over the beef and marinate for 6 hours or overnight.
3. Heat oil and cook beef strips for about 3 minutes. Remove oil and beef from fire.

4. Break spinach into bite-size leaves. Cook spinach for about 3 minutes in the ginger marinade. Drain well. Arrange spinach on platter and place slices of hot meat over spinach.
5. Other green vegetables may be substituted for spinach. Broccoli stalks should be cut in bias strips; broccoli flowers are left whole if small. Cabbage should be sliced. Frozen snow peas or French-style green beans may be used as they are; canned beans or peas should be drained before using.

Cornish Game Hens with Fruited-rice Stuffing
Servings: 8
Exchanges per serving: 1½ fruit A, 3½ fat, 6 meat, 1 bread

Rice Ingredients:
4 cups cooked brown rice
1 17-ounce can apricot halves
1 13¼-ounce can pineapple tidbits
½ cup margarine
1 teaspoon ginger
½ teaspoon allspice
3 tablespoons parsley flakes
¼ teaspoon savory
1 teaspoon salt

Rice Directions:
1. Drain apricots and pineapples and save syrup for glaze. Cut apricot halves into quarters.
2. Melt margarine in large skillet and stir in ginger, allspice, parsley flakes, savory, and salt.
3. Add fruit and cooked rice, tossing lightly to mix.

Hen Ingredients:
8 cornish game hens, approximately 18 ounces each
2 tablespoons salt
2 teaspoons Season-all
½ teaspoon poultry seasoning
½ teaspoon ginger

Hen Directions:
1. Mix salt, Season-all, poultry season, and ginger.
2. Rinse hens, wipe dry, and rub each hen with 1 teaspoon salt-spice mixture.
3. Stuff body of hen loosely with fruited rice stuffing. Band legs together.
4. Place on roasting-pan rack and bake for 75 minutes at 350°.
5. Brush with fruit glaze every 15 to 20 minutes.

Glaze Ingredients:
1½ cups syrup saved from pineapple and apricots
¼ teaspoon salt
¼ teaspoon allspice
½ teaspoon ginger
2 tablespoons butter
2 tablespoons lemon juice

Glaze Directions:
1. Combine butter, lemon juice, salt, allspice, and ginger in a saucepan and bring to a gentle boil.
2. Baste game hens with fruit glaze every 15 to 20 minutes.

Party Chicken
Servings: 6
Exchanges per serving: 5 meat, 2¼ fat

Ingredients:
3 skinned chicken breasts, halved
margarine
6 strips bacon
1 jar dried beef (2½ ounces)
½ pint sour cream (8 ounces)
1 can mushroom soup

Directions:
1. Lightly grease bottom of a broiler pan with margarine.
2. Place a layer of dried-beef slices on bottom of pan.
3. Wrap chicken breasts in bacon strips, tucking strips under breasts as you place breasts onto the dried-beef layer.
4. Mix sour cream and mushroom soup. Spread mixture over meat. Bake in a 275° oven for about 2½ hours or in a 325° oven for 1½ hours. This dish may be prepared ahead of time and refrigerated. it should be baked *uncovered*. The dish may be frozen ahead of time except for sour-cream-mushroom-soup mixture.

Chicken Della Robbia
Servings: 10
Exchanges per serving: 5 fat, 6 meat, 1¾ fruit, ½ bread

Ingredients:
6 tablespoons margarine
2 fryers, 2½ to 3 pounds each (cut up)
2 medium onions, sliced
½ pound mushrooms, sliced
1 cup light or dark raisins
1¼ cups water
4 teaspoons salt
½ teaspoon allspice
½ teaspoon ginger
¼ teaspoon lemon juice
½ teaspoon cloves
¼ cup brown sugar
1 cup walnut halves
4 teaspoons cornstarch
½ cup water
2 cups seedless green grapes
12 maraschino cherries
2 cups orange sections

Directions:
1. Sauté chicken pieces in margarine in Dutch oven.
2. Add onion, mushrooms, raisins, 1¼ cups water, salt, allspice, ginger, brown sugar, lemon juice, and cloves. Mix well.
3. Cover and simmer for 40 minutes, turning occasionally until chicken is tender.
4. Add nuts.
5. Blend cornstarch with ½ cup water. Push chicken to one side. Blend cornstarch with liquid in pot.
6. Heat until smooth and thick. Turn heat down and add fruit.
7. Heat for 2 to 3 minutes.
8. To serve, remove chicken to serving platter and arrange fruit around chicken in a wreath. Drain off sauce to serve over chicken or rice (½ cup rice = 1 bread exchange).

BREAD EXCHANGES

Fortified Peanut-butter-orange Bread
Servings: 9 (1 1" slice per serving)
Exchanges per serving: 2½ bread, 1 meat, 1 fruit, 1¾ fat

Ingredients:
2 cups flour
3 teaspoons baking powder
1 teaspoon salt
1 cup chunky peanut butter
½ cup sugar
2 eggs
1 tablespoon grated orange rind
½ cup orange juice
½ cup milk
1/3 cup nonfat dry milk
1 cup raisins

Directions:
1. Sift flour, baking powder, and salt together.
2. Beat peanut butter, sugar, and eggs with an electric mixer until creamy.
3. Mix nonfat dry milk with orange juice and milk. Add to egg-and-peanut-butter mixture and mix well.
4. Add flour mixture, raisins, and orange rind to peanut-butter mixture, blending until ingredients are moistened.
5. Pour into a greased 9"-x-5"-x-3" loaf pan.
6. Place in 350° oven for 30 minutes, or until toothpick inserted near center comes out clean.
7. Cool in pan or on a rack for 10 minutes. Loosen edges with knife and turn out onto rack to cool completely.
8. Wrap and store overnight before slicing.

Oatmeal-nut Waffles
Servings: 6 (1 waffle per serving)
Exchanges per serving: 2 bread, 2-1/3 fat

Ingredients:
¾ cup whole-wheat flour
1 teaspoon baking powder
¼ teaspoon salt
1 cup 2% milk
1 egg
2 tablespoons melted margarine
1 tablespoon honey
½ cup old-fashioned rolled oats
½ cup finely chopped walnuts or pecans
¼ cup bran flakes or all-bran

Directions:
1. Stir together flour, baking powder, and salt.
2. Add milk, egg, margarine, and honey.
3. Beat until smooth.
4. Stir in oats, nuts, and bran.
5. Cook in hot waffle iron until golden brown.
6. Serve with butter and honey and warm applesauce if desired.

Orange-date Bread
Servings: 10
Exchanges per serving: 3 bread, 1 fruit, 1 fat

Ingredients:
2 cups sifted flour
¾ cup sugar
2 teaspoons baking powder
¼ teaspoon salt
½ cup pecans or walnuts, chopped
½ cup dates, chopped
1 well-beaten egg
3 tablespoons vegetable oil
1 cup orange juice
1¾ tablespoons grated orange peel
½ cup wheat germ

Directions:
1. Sift flour, sugar, baking powder, and salt.
2. Stir in dates and nuts.
3. Mix egg, vegetable oil, orange juice, and orange peel in separate container. Gently stir in wheat germ.
4. Add egg mixture to dry ingredients, stirring just until moistened.
5. Pour into greased 8½"-x-4½"-x-2½" loaf pan and bake for 1 hour at 350°.
6. Let cool 10 to 20 minutes before removing from pan. Flavor is best if loaf stands overnight before serving.

Whole-wheat Fruit Pancakes
Servings: 3 (2 5" pancakes per serving)
Exchanges per serving: 2½ bread, ½ fruit

Ingredients:
½ cup buttermilk
1 egg
1 medium apple, cored, or 1 medium peach or ½ ripe banana
¾ cup whole-wheat flour
1 teaspoon baking powder
½ teaspoon soda
½ teaspoon salt

Directions:
1. Place buttermilk, egg, and fruit pieces in blender. Mix until smooth.
2. Add baking powder, soda, and salt to flour. Then add dry ingredients slowly to mixture in blender. Blend long enough to moisten all ingredients.
3. Preheat griddle on medium-high heat. To test temperature, sprinkle drops of water onto hot surface. If bubbles skitter around, temperature is right.
4. Grease griddle lightly by rubbing with end of margarine stick or use Teflon-coated griddle.
5. Pour batter on griddle. Turn pancakes when bubbles form and edges start to dry.
6. Remove when golden brown and place on platter.

Whole-wheat Muffins
Servings: 3 (2 muffins per serving)
Exchanges per serving: 3 bread, 2/3 meat, 2 fat, 2/3 fruit A

Ingredients:
1 cup whole-wheat flour
½ teaspoon baking powder
2 eggs
2/3 cup 2% milk
¼ stick margarine (⅛ cup)
1 tablespoon honey
¼ cup bran buds
¼ cup raisins

Directions:
1. In medium bowl stir together flour and baking powder.
2. Add eggs, milk, butter, and honey. Stir just until dry ingredients are moistened; do not overmix.
3. Fold in bran buds and raisins.
4. Spoon into greased muffin cups, filling about 2/3 full.
5. Bake in preheated oven at 425° for about 25 minutes, or until golden.

Chalah Bread
Servings: 48 (4 loaves with 12 slices each)
Exchanges per serving: 1½ bread, 1¼ fat

Ingredients:
2 packages active dry yeast
4 teaspoons salt
¾ cup honey
1¾ cups hot water
1¼ cups oil
3 large eggs
8 cups flour
1 egg
poppy seed

Directions:
1. Mix yeast, salt, honey, hot water, and 2 cups of flour in a bowl, beating well with a mixer for at least 5 minutes.
2. Add oil and eggs to flour mixture and continue mixing.
3. Gradually add 4 more cups of flour, mixing well after each addition.
4. Knead in remaining 2 cups of flour until dough is silky but no longer sticky.
5. Place dough in greased bowl, turn over once, cover, and let rise for 1 to 3 hours (bread should more than double).
6. Punch down bread dough and knead to get rid of any bubbles.
7. Cut round of dough into 4 portions. Cut each portion into 3 equal lumps.
8. Knead and roll each lump into a 1"-thick rope.
9. Start in the middle and braid the three ropes, working them out to the end. Repeat for the other lumps of dough.
10. Let 4 braided loaves rise for ½ hour.
11. Beat 1 egg and smear over bread loaves. Sprinkle loaves with poppy seed.
12. Place in 325° to 350° oven for 1 hour.

Finnish Whole-grain Bread
Servings: 8 (1 round loaf)
Exchanges per serving: 2 bread

Ingredients:
1 package active rising yeast
⅛ cup warm water (105 to 115°)
1 cup milk, scalded and cooled to lukewarm
1 teaspoon salt
1 cup whole-wheat flour
Melted butter or margarine

Directions:
1. Dissolve yeast in warm water. Stir in milk, salt, and 1 cup of flour. Gradually add remaining flour and let stand, covered, for 15 minutes.
2. Place dough on greased 10" or 12" pizza pan. Grease fingers and pat dough into circle ¼" to ½" thick. Cover and let rise in warm place until double (about 1 hour).
3. Prick loaf with fork, place in 375° oven, and bake 25 to 30 minutes, or until light brown. Brush with butter while still hot and serve warm, cut into wedges.

Cranberry Bread
Servings: 9 (1 2½" slice per serving)
Exchanges per serving: 3 bread, 2/3 fruit, 1/5 fat

Ingredients:
2 cups flour
1 cup sugar
½ teaspoon soda
½ teaspoon salt
Juice and grated rind of 1 orange
2 teaspoons melted butter
Hot water
1 egg, beaten
1 teaspoon vanilla flavoring
1 cup cranberries, halved
½ cup raisins

Directions:
1. Sift dry ingredients in a large bowl.
2. Place orange juice, grated rind, and melted butter in a measuring cup and add enough hot water to make 1 cup.
3. Stir orange mixture into dry ingredients.
4. Stir in beaten egg and vanilla.
5. Add cranberries and raisins, stirring just until mixed.
6. Pour into greased, floured 9"-x-5"-x-3" loaf pan and place in 350° oven for 1 hour.
7. Let stand 24 hours before serving.

Molasses Cookies
Servings: 20 (2 cookies per serving)
Exchanges per serving: 1½ bread, 1¾ fat

Ingredients:
1 cup sugar
¾ cup margarine
1 egg
¼ cup molasses
¼ teaspoon soda
2 cups flour
½ teaspoon salt
1 teaspoon cinnamon
½ teaspoon nutmeg
1 teaspoon ginger
½ cup sugar (for dipping)

Directions:
1. Blend sugar, margarine, and egg.
2. Add molasses, soda, flour, salt, cinnamon, nutmeg, and ginger. Mix well.
3. Chill dough.
4. Roll into small balls. Dip tops in sugar and place on greased cookie sheet.
5. Place in 400° oven for 8 to 10 minutes.

Sour-cream Pound Cake
Servings: 24 (½"-thick slice per serving)
Exchanges per serving: 1 bread, 1½ fat

Ingredients:
1 cup margarine (2 sticks)
2½ cups sugar
6 eggs
3 cups sifted flour
½ teaspoon salt
¼ teaspoon soda
1 cup sour cream
1 teaspoon vanilla
2 teaspoons lemon flavoring

Directions:
1. Cream margarine and sugar until light.
2. Add eggs 1 at a time, beating thoroughly after each addition.
3. Sift together dry ingredients and add alternately with sour cream to egg mixture, beating until smooth.
4. Add flavoring.
5. Pour into a greased, floured 9" tube pan.
6. Place in 350° oven for 80 minutes.
7. Let stand in pan on rack about 5 minutes before removing to plate.
8. Serve with Cranberry-apple Topping (see below).

Cranberry-apple Topping
Servings: 4
Exchanges per serving: ½ fruit, 1/3 bread

Ingredients:
1 apple (thinly sliced)
1 cup fresh or frozen cranberries
2 tablespoons sugar
⅛ cup water

Directions:
1. Bring water to a boil.
2. Stir in sugar until dissolved.
3. Add apple and cranberries and simmer until cranberries pop (about 3 minutes).
4. Serve over Tizzie's Sour-cream Pound Cake.

Zucchini Bread
Servings: 38 (1 1½" piece per serving)
Exchanges per serving: 1-1/3 bread, 2-1/3 fat

Ingredients:
½ cup wheat germ
1/3 cup sesame seed
3 eggs
1 cup salad oil

1 cup brown sugar
1 cup granulated sugar
3 teaspoons maple syrup or 1½ teaspoons almond flavoring
2 cups grated zucchini
2½ cups flour
2 teaspoons soda
2 teaspoons salt
½ teaspoon baking powder
1 cup chopped nuts

Directions:
1. In separate pan toast wheat germ and sesame seed at 300° for 5 minutes.
2. Beat eggs and add salad oil, brown sugar, granulated sugar, and flavoring. Beat again until foamy.
3. Stir in 2 cups grated zucchini.
4. In separate bowl mix flour, soda, salt, and baking powder.
5. Add chopped nuts to flour mixture and stir well.
6. Add flour mixture to egg mixture. Stir just to blend.
7. Pour into 2 9½"-x-5¼" loaf pans.
8. Sprinkle with toasted sesame seed and bake at 300° for 1 hour.
9. Cool for 10 minutes before removing from pan.
10. This bread freezes well.

Green Peas with Mushrooms
Servings: 6
Exchanges per serving: ½ vegetable, 1 bread

Ingredients:
2 10½-ounce packages frozen green peas
½ onion, chopped
1 4-ounce can mushrooms
¼ cup water

Directions:
1. Place water in saucepan.
2. Drain liquid from mushrooms into saucepan.
3. Add chopped onion and bring to a rapid boil.
4. Add green peas and mushrooms, reduce heat, and simmer for 3 to 5 minutes, or until peas are fork tender.

New Potatoes
Servings: 4 (4 small potatoes per serving)
Exchanges per serving: 2 bread B, 1½ fat

Ingredients:
16 very small new potatoes
4 cups water
2 tablespoons butter

Directions:
1. Wash potatoes thoroughly, removing any imperfections.
2. Place potatoes and water in large saucepan and bring to rapid boil. Boil 3 to 5 minutes. Drain potatoes and place in 9" pie plate or 9"-x-9" cake pan. Place small dab of butter on each potato.
3. Place in 425° oven for 60 minutes, turning once to apply butter to undersides.
4. Remove to serving dish and serve while warm.

Saffron Rice with Peas and Mushrooms
Servings: 6 to 8 (1 cup per serving)
Exchanges per serving: 2 bread, 3 fat

Ingredients:
½ stick margarine
½ cup slivered almonds
1 cup rice
2 tablespoons chopped onions
1 cup chopped green pepper
1 4-ounce can mushrooms, stems and pieces
1 10-ounce package frozen green peas
¼ teaspoon saffron pieces
¼ teaspoon black pepper
1½ teaspoons salt
2½ cups water

Directions:
1. Melt margarine in skillet. Add almonds, rice, and onions and cook over low heat stirring until rice is delicately browned and onions are transparent.
2. Add remaining ingredients, cover skillet, and bring to a boil.
3. Reduce heat and simmer about 25 minutes.
4. Remove from heat and keep covered until serving time.

Swart's Baked Beans
Servings: 8 to 10
Exchanges per serving: 1 bread, 2½ meat

Ingredients:
1 cup red kidney beans
½ cup navy beans
½ cup pinto beans
2 strips bacon
1 teaspoon salt
2 pounds lean ground beef
2 medium onions, chopped
2 medium bell peppers, chopped
2 pimento peppers, chopped
¼ cup sweet-pickle relish

¼ cup molasses or syrup
3 tablespoons chili powder
2 tablespoons vinegar
1 teaspoon cumin
1 teaspoon Worcestershire sauce
Dash of tabasco or cayenne pepper if desired
1 cup Kraft hickory-smoked barbecue sauce

Directions:
1. Soak beans overnight in 6 cups water, then cook with bacon and salt for 1½ to 2 hours. Or do not soak beans but pressure-cook them with 5 cups water at 15 pounds of pressure for 90 minutes.
2. Brown meat in large skillet, add onions and peppers, and cook until tender. Drain off excess grease.
3. Add pimento peppers, relish, molasses, chili powder, vinegar, cumin, Worcestershire sauce, and tabasco or cayenne pepper if desired to meat mixture. Stir well.
4. Pour meat mixture into beans and mix well. Add 1 cup Kraft hickory-smoked barbecue sauce and mix thoroughly.
5. Place beans in 325° oven for 1 hour, stirring occasionally to prevent excessive drying on top.
6. 5 cans of Campbells ranch-style beans may be substituted for the bean mixture described above. If canned beans are used, drain excess liquid from beans before proceeding with recipe.

FAT EXCHANGE

Sesame-seed Snack
Servings: 16
Exchanges per serving: 2 fat, ¼ bread

Ingredients:
2 cups sesame seeds
4 to 5 tablespoons honey
Wheat germ, as needed

Directions:
1. Mix sesame seeds and honey.
2. Add wheat germ to allow for easy handling.
3. Press mixture into a 9" buttered pan.
4. Allow to harden for 24 hours.
5. Cut into 16 equal servings.

APPENDIX I.
DESIGNING A MEAL-PATTERN CHART

1. Establish a desired calorie level, following the suggestions in chapter 7.
2. Place the number of calories in the blank at the top of the page and in the double-line box at the lower-right corner of the grid.
3. Consult the recommended-minmum-daily-totals line to determine the exchanges that must be included in any day's snacks and meals. Decide whether these nucleus items will be in meals or snacks. For example, the four milk exchanges might be included as one at breakfast and one at lunch and dinner.
4. Place the nucleus items on the meal-pattern chart by entering the number of exchanges per meal or snack in the appropriate columns.
5. Referring to the top of the chart (kcal/exchanges), multiply the number of exchanges by the number of calories per exchange and enter the calories in the column to the right of the exchange. For example, one skim-milk exchange at breakfast would mean 80 calories in the appropriate column, or two vegetable exchanges for lunch would mean 50 calories in the appropriate column.
6. Once the recommended (nucleus) exchanges have been placed on the chart, continue to enter any desired *extra* calories until the calorie total is approached or reached.
7. Total the milk, vegetable, fruit, bread, meat, and fat columns. Add these totals to determine the total number of calories planned for the entire day.
8. If the calorie load exceeds the desired maximum, delete the necessary number of exchanges. If the calorie load falls below the desired maximum, add exchanges until the maximum level is reached. Remember: *Do not subtract exchanges from the nucleus group!*
9. Double-check your figures by adding across the chart, writing the total calories for each meal and snack in the column at the far right, totaling these numbers, and recording the day's actual calorie total in the appropriate box.

DAILY MEAL PATTERN FOR _____ CALORIE PRENATAL DIET

	MILK				VEGETABLE				FRUIT			BREAD			MEAT				FAT		Total
	A 80	B 125	C 170	Milk Kcal Per Meal Or Snack	A 25	B 25	C 25	Vegetable Kcal Per Meal Or Snack	A 40	B 40	Fruit Kcal Per Meal Or Snack	A 70	B 70	Bread Kcal Per Meal Or Snack	A 55	B 77	C 100	Meat Kcal Per Meal Or Snack	45	Fat Kcal Per Meal Or Snack	Kcal Per Meal Or Snack
Breakfast																					
Mid - morning Snack																					
Lunch																					
Afternoon Snack																					
Dinner																					
Evening Snack																					
Actual Daily Totals Per Exchange																					
Recommended Minimum Daily Totals	4			varies 320-680	2				1		75	1		40	3		1	280	8 - 9		varies 495-900	as needed to meet calorie requirements	Maximum [ ] Calories

APPENDIX II.
RECOMMENDED READING

Nutrition*

Nutrition During Pregnancy and Lactation, California Dept. of Health, Sacramento, California, 1975.

Maternal Nutrition and the Course of Pregnancy, Committee on Maternal Nutrition, Food and Nutrition Board, National Research Council, National Academy of Science, Washington, D.C., 1970.

Nutrition in Maternal Health Care, Committee on Nutrition, American College of Obstetricians and Gynecologists, Chicago, Illinois, 1974.

Recommended Dietary Allowances, Food and Nutrition Board of National Research Council, National Academy of Science, Washington D.C. 1974.

White Paper on Infant Feeding Practices, Citizens' Committee on Infant Nutrition, Center for Science in the Public Interest, Washington, D.C., 1974.

Prenatal**

Preparation for Childbirth (a Lamaze guide), Donna and Roger Ewy, Signet, 1970.

Six Practical Lessons for an Easier Childbirth, Elisabeth Bing, Grosset and Dunlap, New York, 1967.

Childbirth Without Fear, Grantly Dick-Read, Harper and Row, New York, 1960.

Breast Feeding***

The Womanly Art of Breastfeeding, La Leche League International, Franklin Park, Illinois.

Nursing Your Baby, Karen Pryor, Pocket Books, New York, 1973.

Preparation for Breastfeeding, Donna and Roger Ewy, Doubleday, New York, 1975.

Let's Have Healthy Children, Adelle Davis, Signet, New York, 1972.

Exercise

Write to ASOP and ICEA (see **) for additional prenatal exercises. Also see prenatal publications listed above. Your doctor shoud have available pamphlets such as "Rapid Post Natal Figure Recovery" by Constance Reed, Ortho Pharamceutical Corporation, 1967. This particular pamphlet stresses exercises to tone up and/or slim down specific body areas.

*For extensive reading on prenatal nutrition see *Annotated Bibliography on Maternal Nutrition*, Committee on Maternal Nutrition, Food and Nutrition Board, National Research Council, National Academy of Science, U.S. Department of Health, Education and Welfare, Washington, D.C., 1970.

**For information on the availability of childbirth-education classes in your area write to International Childbirth Education Association (ICEA), Box 5852, Milwaukee, Wisconsin 53220 or The American Society for Psychoprophylaxis in Obstetrics (ASPO), 7 West 96 Street, New York, N.Y. 10025.

***For extensive information on all aspects of breast feeding write to La Leche League International, Inc., 9616 Minneapolis Avenue, Franklin Park, Illinois 60131.

BIBLIOGRAPHY

The following books and articles are the primary sources for this book. No attempt has been made to devise a comprehensive bibliography on prenatal and postpartum nutrition, since the sources are far too numerous to be listed in a book such as this.

Preface

Asling, C.W., et al., "The Development of Cleft Palate Resulting from Maternal Pteroylglutamic [folic] Acid Deficiency During the Latter Half of Gestation in Rats," *Surgical and Gynecological Obstetrics*, III, 1960, pp. 19-28.

Hurley, L.S. and H. Sevenerton, "Congenital Malformation Resulting from Zinc Deficiency in Rats," *Proceedings Soc. Exp. Biol. Med.*, Vol. 123, 1966, pp. 692-696.

Lee, C.J. and B.F. Chow, "Protein Metabolism in the Offspring of Underfed Mother Rats," *Journal of Nutrition*, Vol. 87, 1965, pp. 439-443.

Zamenhof, S., E. VanMarthens, and F.L. Margolis, "DNA [cell number] and Protein in Neonatal Brain: Alteration by Material Dietary Protein Restriction" *Science*, Vol. 160, 1968, 322-323.

Chapter 1

Antonov, A.M., "Children Born During the Seige of Leningrad in 1942," *Journal of Pediatrics*, Vol. 30, 1947, pp. 250-259.

Brandt, M.B., "Nutrition in Pregnancy," *Clinical Obstetrics and Gynecology*, Vol. 6, September 1963, pp. 604-618.

Burke, B.S., et al., "The Influence of Nutrition Upon the Condition of the Infant at Birth," *Journal of Nutrition*, Vol. 26, 1943, pp. 569-583.

Committee on Maternal Nutrition, Food and Nutrition Board, National Research Council, *Maternal Nutrition and the Course of Pregnancy*, National Academy of Sciences, Washington, D.C., 1970.

Coursin, David B., "Maternal Nutrition and the Offspring's Development," *Nutrition Today*, Vol. 8, March/April 1973, pp. 12-18.

Davis, Adelle, *Let's Have Healthy Children*. New York: New American Library, 1972.

Ebbs, J.H., F.F. Tisdall, and W.A. Scott, "The Influence of Prenatal Diet on the Mother and Child," *Journal of Nutrition*, Vol. 22, 1941, pp. 515+.

Gold, Edwin M., editor. *Proceedings of the National Conference for the Prevention of Mental Retardation Through Improved Maternity Care*, March 27-29, 1968, Washington, D.C.

Jance, Virginia C., "Maternal Nutrition in the 1970's," Part 1, *Food and Nutrition News*, National Livestock and Meat Board, Chicago, Illinois, Vol. 46, December/January 1974-75, pp. 1, 4.

Kasius, R.V. et al., "Maternal and Newborn Nutrition Studies at Philadelphia Lying-in Hospital. Newborn Studies: I, Size and Growth of Babies of Mothers Receiving Nutrient Supplements," *Milbank Memorial Fund Quarterly*, Vol. 33, 1955, pp. 230-245.

Lechtig, A. et al., "Effect of Food Supplementation During Pregnancy on Birthweight," *Pediatrics*, Vol. 56, October 1975, pp. 508-520.

McGanity, W.J. et al., "The Vanderbilt Study on Maternal and Infant Nutrition. V. Description and Outcome of Obstetric Sample," *American J. Obstet Gynecol*, Vol. 67, 1954, pp. 491-500.

McGanity, W.J. et al., "The Vanderbilt Study of Maternal and Infant Nutrition. VI. Relationship of Obstetric Performance and Nutrition," *American Journal Obstet Gynecol.*, Vol. 67, 1954, pp. 501-527.

Mayer, Jean, "Some Aspects of the Relation of Nutrition and Pregnancy," *Human Nutrition: Its Physiological, Medical and Social Aspects*, Charles C. Thomas: Springfield, Illinois, 1972, pp. 206-215.

Mayer, Jean, "White House Conference on Food, Nutrition and Health, 1969," *Human Nutrition: Its Physiological, Medical and Social Aspects*, Charles C. Thomas: Springfield, Illinois, 1972, pp. 639-645.

"Search and Save Program Spreading for Mothers-to-Be," Associated Press Release, *Bozeman Daily Chronicle*, Thursday, October 7, 1976, p. 13.

Stare, Frederick J. and Margaret McWilliams. *Living Nutrition*, John Wiley & Sons, Inc., N.Y., 1973.

Williams, Roger J. *Physicians' Handbook of Nutritional Science*, Charles C. Thomas, Springfield, Illinois, 1975.

Williams, Sue Rodwell. *Nutrition and Diet Therapy*, C.V. Mosby Company: St. Louis, 1969.

Chapter 2

Brandt, M.B., "Nutrition in Pregnancy," *Clinical Obstetrics and Gynecology*, Vol. 6, September 1963, pp. 604-618.

California Department of Health, *Nutrition During Pregnancy and Lactation*, California Department of Health, Sacramento, California, 1975.

Clinical Obstetrics, Philadelphia: J.B. Lippincott, 1953.

Committee on Maternal Nutrition, Food and Nutrition Board, National Research Council, *Maternal Nutrition and the Course of Pregnancy*, National Academy of Sciences, Washington, D.C., 1970.

Committee on Maternal Nutrition, Food and Nutrition Board, National Research Council, National Academy of Science, *Maternal Nutrition and the Course of Pregnancy: Summary Report*, HEW, Washington, D.C., 1970.

Committee on Nutrition, American College of Obstetricians and Gynecologists, *Nutrition in Maternal Health Care*, American College of Obstetricians and Gynecologists, Chicago, Illinois, 1974.

Coursin, David B., "Maternal Nutrition and the Offspring's Development," *Nutrition Today*, Vol. 8, March/April 1973, pp. 12-18.

Hytten, F.E. and A.M. Thompson, "Maternal Physiological Adjustments," *Maternal Nutrition and the Course of Pregnancy*, Committee on Maternal Nutrition, Food and Nutrition Board, National Research Council, National Academy of Science, Washington, D.C., 1970, pp. 41-73.

Jance, Virginia C., "Maternal Nutrition in the 1970's," Part 1, *Food and Nutrition News*, National Livestock and Meat Board, Chicago, Illinois, Vol. 46, December/January 1974-75, pp. 1, 4.

Krause, Fred J., "How to Prevent Mental Retardation," *Parents*, Vol. 51, August 1976, pp. 72+.

Mayer, Jean, et al., "Management of Weight in Pregnancy," *Postgraduate Medicine*, Vol. 48, July, 1970.

"Metabolic Adaptations to Pregnancy," *Nutrition Reviews*, Vol. 32, September 1974, pp. 270-272.

"Starvation in Pregnancy: Metabolic Changes," *Nutrition Reviews*, Vol. 31, March 1973, pp. 82-83.

Winick, Myron, "Preventing Growth-Retarded Children," *Current Prescribing*, July 1976, pp. 43-47.

Chapter 3

California Department of Health, *Nutrition During Pregnancy and Lactation*, California Department of Health, Sacramento, California, 1975.

Committee on Maternal Nutrition, Food and Nutrition Board, National Research Council, National Academy of Science, *Maternal Nutrition and the Course of Pregnancy: Summary Report*, HEW, Washington, D.C., 1970.

Committee on Nutrition, American College of Obstetricians and Gynecologists, *Nutrition in Maternal Health Care*, American College of Obstetricians and Gynecologists, Chicago, Illinois, 1974.

Erhard, Darla, "The New Vegetarians—Part One—Vegetarianism and Its Medical Consequences," *Nutrition Today*, Vol. 8, November/December, 1973, pp. 4-12.

Erhard, Darla, "The New Vegetarians—Part Two—The Zen Macrobiotic Movement and Other Cults Based on Vegetarianism," *Nutrition Today*, Vol. 9, January/February, 1974, pp. 20-27.

Gold, Edwin M., editor, *Proceedings of the National Conference for the Prevention of Mental Retardation Through Improved Maternity Care*, March 27-29, 1968, Washington, D.C.

Jance, Virginia C., "Maternal Nutrition in the 1970's," Part II, *Food and Nutrition News*, National Livestock and Meat Board, Chicago, Illinois, Vol. 46, February 1975, pp. 1, 4.

Mayer, Jean, et al., "Nutrition Related Problems in Pregnancy," *Postgraduate Medicine*, Vol. 48, October, 1974.

Williams, Sue Rodwell. Nutrition and Diet Therapy, C.V. Mosby Company: St. Louis, 1969.

The Working Group, "Relation of Nutrition to Fetal Growth and Development," *Maternal Nutrition and the Course of Pregnancy*, Committee on Maternal Nutrition, National Research Council, National Academy of Sciences, Washington, D.C., 1970, pp. 110-138.

Chapter 4

Berland, Theodore and the editors of *Consumer Guide, Rating the Diets*, Chicago: Rand, McNally and Company, 1974.

California Department of Health, *Nutrition During Pregnancy and Lactation*, California Department of Health, Sacramento, California, 1975.

"The Caloric Cost of Pregnancy," *Nutrition Reviews*, Vol. 31, June 1973, pp. 177-179.

Cheek, Donald B., "The Fetus," *Fetal and Postnatal Cellular Growth*, New York: John Wiley and Sons, 1975.

Cheek, Donald B., "Maternal Nutritional Restriction and Fetal Brain Growth," in *Fetal and Postnatal Cellular Growth*, New York: John Wiley and Sons, 1975.

Committee on Maternal Nutrition, Food and Nutrition Board, National Research Council, National Academy of Science, *Maternal Nutrition and the Course of Pregnancy: Summary Report*, HEW, Washington, D.C., 1970.

Committee on Nutrition, American College of Obstetricians and Gynecologists, *Nutrition in Maternal Health Care*, American College of Obstetricians and Gynecologists, Chicago, Illinois, 1974.

Coursin, David B., "Maternal Nutrition and the Offspring's Development," *Nutrition Today*, Vol. 8, March/April 1973, pp. 12-18.

Felig, P., "Maternal and Fetal Fuel Homeostasis," *American Journal of Clinical Nutrition*, Vol. 26, September, 1973, pp. 998-1005.

Felig, P. and V. Lynch, "Starvation in Human Pregnancy: Hypoglycemia, Hypoinsulinemia, and Hyperketonemia," *Science*, Vol. 170, November, 1970, pp. 990-992.

Food and Nutrition Board, National Research Council, *Recommended Dietary Allowances*, National Academy of Sciences Publication #1694, Washington, D.C., 1968.

Food and Nutrition Board, National Research Council, *Recommended Dietary Allowances*, 8th ed., National Academy of Sciences, Washington, D.C., 1974.

Stare, Frederick J. and Margaret McWilliams, *Living Nutrition*, John Wiley & Sons, Inc.: New York, 1973.

Williams, Sue Rodwell. *Nutrition and Diet Therapy*, C.V. Mosby Company: St. Louis, 1969.

Chapter 5

California Department of Health, *Nutrition During Pregnancy and Lactation*, California Department of Health, Sacramento, California, 1975.

Cochran, W.A., "Overnutrition in Prenatal and Neonatal Life: A Problem," *Canadian Medical Association Journal*, Vol. 93, 1965, pp. 893-899.

Committee on Maternal Nutrition, Food and Nutrition Board, National Research Council, National Academy of Science, *Maternal Nutrition and the Course of Pregnancy: Summary Report*, HEW, Washington, D.C., 1970.

Committee on Nutrition, American College of Obstetricians and Gynecologists, *Nutrition in Maternal Health Care*, American College of Obstetricians and Gynecologists, Chicago, Illinois, 1974.

Corrigan, J.J., Jr. and F.I. Marcus, "Coagulopathy Associated with Vitamin E Ingestion," *Journal of American Medical Association*, Vol. 230, 1974, pp. 1300-1301.

Food and Nutrition Board, National Research Council, *Recommended Dietary Allowances*, National Academy of Sciences Publication #1694, Washington, D.C., 1968.

Food and Nutrition Board, National Research Council, *Recommended Dietary Allowances*, 8th ed., National Academy of Sciences, Washington, D.C., 1974.

Hytten, F.E. and A.M. Thompson, "Maternal Physiological Adjustments," *Maternal Nutrition and the Course of Pregnancy*, Committee on Maternal Nutrition, Food and Nutrition Board, National Research Council, National Academy of Science, Washington, D.C., 1970, pp. 41-73.

Mayer, Jean, "Some Aspects of the Relation of Nutrition and Pregnancy," *Human Nutrition: Its Physiological, Medical and Social Aspects*, Charles C. Thomas: Springfield, Illinois, 1972, pp. 206-215.

"Too Much Nutrition Harmful," Associated Press Release from Pullman, Washington, *Bozeman Daily Chronicle*, October 31, 1976.

Williams, Sue Rodwell. *Nutrition and Diet Therapy*, C.V. Mosby Company: St. Louis, 1969.

World Health Organization Technical Report Series 302, 1965.

Chapter 6

Albanese, Anthony A., "Nutritional Aspects of Bone Loss" [2 parts] *Food and Nutrition News*, Vol. 47, #1, #2, October-November 1975, December-January 1975, pp. 1, 4.

Birch, William G. with Donna Z. Meilach. *A Doctor Discusses Pregnancy*. Budlong Press Company: Chicago, Illinois, 1975.

Brandt, M.B., "Nutrition in Pregnancy," *Clinical Obstetrics and Gynecology*, Vol. 6, September 1963, pp. 604-618.

California Department of Health, *Nutrition During Pregnancy and Lactation*, California Department of Health, Sacramento, California, 1975.

Committee on Maternal Nutrition, Food and Nutrition Board, National Research Council, National Academy of Science, *Maternal Nutrition and the Course of Pregnancy: Summary Report*, HEW, Washington, D.C., 1970.

Committee on Nutrition, American College of Obstetricians and Gynecologists, *Nutrition in Maternal Health Care*, American College of Obstetricians and Gynecologists, Chicago, Illinois, 1974.

Coursin, David B., "Maternal Nutrition and the Offspring's Development," *Nutrition Today*, Vol. 8, March/April 1973, pp. 12-18.

Cullen, Robert W. and Susan M. Oace, *Journal of Nutrition Education*, Vol. 8, July/September 1976, pp. 101-102.

Food and Nutrition Board, National Research Council, *Recommended Dietary Allowances*, National Academy of Sciences Publication #1694, Washington, D.C., 1968.

Food and Nutrition Board, National Research Council, *Recommended Dietary Allowances*, 8th ed., National Academy of Sciences, Washington, D.C., 1974.

Hambridge, K.M., et al., "Zinc Nutrition of Preschool Children in the Denver Head Start Program," *American Journal of Clinical Nutrition*, Vol. 29, 1976, pp. 734+.

Holvey, David N. and John H. Talbott, editors, *The Merck Manual of Diagnosis and Therapy*, 12th edition, Merck Sharp and Dohme Research Laboratories: Rathway, New Jersey, 1972.

"Iodine Fortification and Thyrotoxicosis," *Nutrition Reviews*, Vol. 28, August 1970, pp. 212-214.

Krehl, Willard A., "Selenium—the Maddening Mineral," *Nutrition Today*, Vol. 5, Winter 1970, pp. 26-32.

Lutwak, Leo, "Dietary Calcium and the Reversal of Bone Demineralization," *Nutrition News*, Vol. 37, February 1974, pp. 1, 4.

Staff Report, "Iodized Salt," *Nutrition Today*, Spring 1969, pp. 22-25.

Williams, Sue Rodwell, *Nutrition and Diet Therapy*, C.V. Mosby Company: St. Louis, 1969.

Chapter 7

California Department of Health, *Nutrition During Pregnancy and Lactation*, California Department of Health, Sacramento, California, 1975.

Cinnamon, Pamela and M.A. Swanson, *Everything You Always Wanted To Know (But were Unable to Find Out) About Exchange Values for Foods*, Moscow, Idaho: University Cities Diabetes Education Program, 1973.

Exchange List for Meal Planning, American Diabetes Association, 1976.

Food and Nutrition Board, National Research Council, *Recommended Dietary Allowances*, 8th ed., National Academy of Sciences, Washington, D.C., 1974.

Gormican, Annette. *Controlling Diabetes with Diet*, Springfield, Illinois: Charles C. Thomas, 1971.

Williams, Sue Rodwell, *Nutrition and Diet Therapy*, C.V. Mosby Company: St. Louis, 1969.

Chapter 8

Birch, William G. with Donna Z. Meilach, *A Doctor Discusses Pregnancy*, Budlong Press Company: Chicago, 1975.

Brandt, M.B., "Nutrition in Pregnancy," *Clinical Obstetrics and Gynecology*, Vol. 6, September 1963, pp. 604-618.

Committee on Maternal Nutrition, Food and Nutrition Board, National Research Council, National Academy of Science, *Maternal Nutrition and the Course of Pregnancy: Summary Report*, HEW, Washington, D.C., 1970.

Fitzpatrick, Elise, J.E. Nicholson, and Sharon P. Reader, *Maternity Nursing*, 11th ed., Philadelphia: J.B. Lippincott, 1966.

Fugo, Nicholas W., "Management of Common Problems of Prenatal Care," *Clinical Obstetrics and Gynecology*, Vol. 6, September 1963, pp. 627-638.

Holvey, David N. and John H. Talbott, editors, *The Merck Manual of Diagnosis and Therapy*, 12th edition, Merck Sharp and Dohme Research Laboratories: Rathway, New Jersey, 1972.

Reuben, David, *The Save Your Life Diet*, Ballantine Books: New York, 1975.

Robinson, Corinne H., *Fundamentals of Normal Nutrition*. MacMillan Company: New York, 1968.

Williams, Sue Rodwell, *Nutrition and Diet Therapy*, C.V. Mosby Company: St. Louis, 1969.

Chapter 9

Arena, Jay M., M.D., "Contamination of the Ideal Food," *Nutrition Today*, Vol. 5, Winter 1970, pp. 2-8.

California Department of Health, *Nutrition During Pregnancy and Lactation*, California Department of Health, Sacramento, California, 1975.

Citizens' Committee on Infant Nutrition, *White Paper on Infant Feeding Practices*, Washington, D.C.: Center for Science in the Public Interest, 1974.

Cochrane, W.A., "Overnutrition in Prenatal and Neonatal Life: A Problem," *Canadian Medical Association Journal*, Vol. 93, 1965, pp. 893-899.

"Commentary on Breast-Feeding and Infant Formulas, Including Proposed Standards for Formulas," *Nutrition Reviews*, Vol. 32, August 1976, pp. 248-256.

Committee on Nutrition, American College of Obstetricians and Gynecologists, *Nutrition in Maternal Health Care*, American College of Obstetricians and Gynecologists, Chicago, Illinois, 1974.

Fitzpatrick, Elise, J.E. Nicholson, and Sharon P. Reader, *Maternity Nursing*, 11th ed., Philadelphia: J.B. Lippincott, 1966.

Gerrard, John W., "Breast-Feeding: Second Thoughts," *Pediatrics*, Vol. 54, December 1974, pp. 757-764.

Hall, Barbara, "Changing Composition of Human Milk and Early Development of an Appetite Control," *Lancet*, April 5, 1975, pp. 779-781.

Hytten, F.E. and A.M. Thompson, "Maternal Physiological Adjustments," *Maternal Nutrition and the Course of Pregnancy*, Committee on Maternal Nutrition, Food and Nutrition Board, National Research Council, National Academy of Science, Washington, D.C., 1970, pp. 41-73.

Klaus, Marshall H. and John H. Kennell, *Maternal Infant Bonding*, St. Louis: C.V. Mosby Company, 1976.

La Leche League International, *The Womanly Art of Breastfeeding*, La Leche League International, Franklin Park, Illinois, 1963.

Mayer, Jean, "Baby Foods—A New Look at Old Formulas," *Family Health*, Vol. 8, October 1976, pp. 38-40+.

Mayer, Jean, "Is Breast-Feeding Coming Back," *Human Nutrition: Its Physiological, Medical and Social Aspects*, Charles C. Thompson: Springfield, Illinois, 1972, pp. 229-231.

Mayer, Jean, "The Dimensions of Human Hunger," *Scientific American*, Vol. 235, September 1976, pp. 40-49.

Mayer, Jean, "Nutrition and Lactation," *Human Nutrition: Its Physiological, Medical and Social Aspects*, Charles C. Thompson: Springfield, Illinois, 1972, pp. 232-241.

Mayer, Jean, et al., "Management of Weight in Pregnancy," *Postgraduate Medicine*, Vol. 48, July 1970; "Metabolic Adaptations to Pregnancy," *Nutrition Reviews*, Vol. 32, September 1974, pp. 270-272.

"The Uniqueness of Human Milk," *American Journal of Clinical Nutrition*, Vol. 24, August 1971. (Reprints available at $1.75 each.)

Williams, Sue Rodwell, *Nutrition and Diet Therapy*, C.V. Mosby Company: St. Louis, 1969.

Chapter 10

Arena, Jay M., M.D., "Contamination of the Ideal Food," *Nutrition Today*, Vol. 5, Winter 1970, pp. 2-8.

California Department of Health, *Nutrition During Pregnancy and Lactation*, California Department of Health, Sacramento, California, 1975.

Committee on Nutrition, American College of Obstetricians and Gynecologists, *Nutrition in Maternal Health Care*, American College of Obstetricians and Gynecologists, Chicago, Illinois, 1974.

Davis, Adelle, *Let's Have Healthy Children*, New York, NAL, 1972.

Food and Nutrition Board, National Research Council, *Recommended Dietary Allowances*, National Academy of Sciences Publication #1694, Washington, D.C., 1968.

Food and Nutrition Board, National Research Council, *Recommended Dietary Allowances*, 8th ed., National Academy of Sciences, Washington, D.C., 1974.

Gerrard, John W., "Breast-Feeding: Second Thoughts," *Pediatrics*, Vol. 54, December 1974, pp. 757-764.

Giles, C. and E. Shuttleworth, "Megaloblastic Anemia of Pregnancy and the Puerperium," *Lancet*, 7061, 1958, pp. 1341+.

Hahn, P. and O. Koldorsky, "Late Effects of Premature Weaning on Blood Cholesterol Levels in Adult Rats," *Nutrition Report International*, Vol. 13, 1976, pp. 87+.

Mayer, Jean, "Baby Foods—A New Look at Old Formulas," *Family Health*, Vol. 8, October 1976, pp. 38-40+.

Mayer, Jean, "Nutrition and Lactation," *Human Nutrition: Its Physiological, Medical and Social Aspects*, Charles C. Thompson: Springfield, Illinois, 1972, pp. 232-241.

Mayer, Jean, et al., "Nutrition Related Problems in Pregnancy," *Postgraduate Medicine*, Vol. 48, October, 1970.

Parkins, Dr. Frederick, "Prescribing Fluoride Supplements for Home Use," *Fluorides: An Update for Dental Practice*, American Academy of Pedodontics, Medcom: New York, 1976.

"PBB's Effects Noted," *New York Times*, August 12, 20:1, 20:6, August 15, IV, 6:1.

"PCB's and All That," *Leaven*, September-October 1976, p. 26.

Pryor, Karen, *Nursing Your Baby*, Pocket Books: New York, 1973.

Thomson, A.M. et al., "The Energy Cost of Human Lactation," *British Journal of Nutrition*, Vol. 24, 1970, pp. 565-572.

Tompson, Marian, "PCB's in Mother's Milk," *La Leche League News*, Vol. 18, November-December 1976, pp. 90-92.

Wei, Stephen, Head of Department of Pedodontics, University of Iowa, in phone conversation with Dr. George Carson, Pedodontist, Bozeman, Montana, November 1976.

Williams, Sue Rodwell, *Nutrition and Diet Therapy*, C.V. Mosby Company: St. Louis, 1969.

Chapter 11

California Department of Health, *Nutrition During Pregnancy and Lactation*, California Department of Health, Sacramento, California, 1975.

Food and Nutrition Board, National Research Council, *Recommended Dietary Allowances*, 8th ed., National Academy of Sciences, Washington, D.C., 1974.

La Leche League Internatinal, *The Womanly Art of Breastfeeding*, La Leche League International, Franklin Park, Illinois, 1963.

Williams, Sue Rodwell, *Nutrition and Diet Therapy*, C.V. Mosby Company: St. Louis, 1969.

INDEX